Reviews for *Asian Longevity Secrets*

This book provides a distinctive view of holistic health and is well worth a careful reading.

–*Dr. David Heber, Director, UCLA Center for Human Nutrition*

This is a remarkable and well-written book by a healer who has been thoroughly trained in both traditional "Chinese" medicine as well as modern "Western" medicine. Although some of the ideas are controversial and may seem strange to the non-oriental reader, they are clearly presented, and if read without prejudice, easily understood. I recommend it highly to anyone who enjoys fresh and stimulating new ideas.

–*Novera Herbert Spector, Prof., Physiology, Neuroscience, Microbiology, Gerontology and Psychiatry at 5 Medical Schools in USA and Europe*

A landmark book for anyone who is seriously seeking to achieve longevity. The information and program offered is complete in scope and readily applicable. It goes beyond current methods, combining 5,000 years of time-proven methods with modern scientific research.

–*Harold Udelman, M.D. (Psychiatrist), President, Biomedical Stress Research Foundation*

This is a very unique book that delivers important information. It is a combination of east and west, vibratory and biochemical, alternative and conventional, combining the best of all. Some of my patients have used the protocol and herbs with great success. I highly recommend it be read with an open mind.

–*Tom Grade, M.D. (pain management & anesthesiologist)*

I almost lost my life to late-stage ovarian cancer. As it stood I had almost no chance for survival. I entrusted my life to a team of renowned Cancer Specialists, and to the breakthrough protocols. Together they have given me a second chance at life! I truly believe that without Ping's protocols I would not be here today. And this is not just my opinion. My physician, a very well-known authority, concurred with Ping's recommended protocols for me, and I began in earnest! What is so impressive about Ping's protocols is that they build you up and work with modern medicine to increase your strength and health, or, as in my case, strongly contribute to a seriously ill patient's chance for survival. As a cancer survivor, I strongly urge everyone to get regular checkups, read this breakthrough book, and live the protocols starting today, for this day, and... every day is truly precious!

–*Julie Larson-Boyd, President of Mitogenesis Corporation*

Asian Longevity Secrets

Seven Breakthrough Steps
to Youthful Health and Vitality

Ping Wu, M.D., and Taichi Tzu, Ph.D.

PingClinic Publishing

Copyright © 2003 by PingClinic, LLC
All rights reserved under International and
Pan-American Copyright conventions
Published in the United States by
PingClinic Publishing, a division of
PingClinic, LLC
P.O. Box 806, Laguna Beach, CA 92651-806
The United States of America
www.pingclinic.com
For Book Orders 1-866-608-1717

ISBN   0-9709887-9-6
Library of Congress Control Number   2003091329

Printed in the United States of America

The book is not intended to replace medical advice
or be a substitute for a physician.
We advise the reader to consult with a physician before
beginning any program of this book. The authors
disclaim any liability, personal or otherwise, resulting
from the procedures in this book.

DEDICATED TO A HEALTHIER
AND MORE SPIRITUALLY
DEVELOPED MANKIND

CONTENTS

ACKNOWLEDGMENTS

This book is a result of lifelong learning from our own experience, study, and research as well as from fellow scientists and doctors.

In particular, we are grateful for the opportunity to have visited and worked with some of the first-rate scientists in China: Dr. Liu Fenjun, Beijing Dadao Herbal Medicine Research Institute; Dr. Xie Bonghe, Hengxing Cancer Research Institute; Professor Cheng Xinong, Chinese Academy of Sciences; Dr. Kang Xisheng, Beijing Medical University Hospital; Dr. Xiao Zhengquan, China Academy of Traditional Chinese Medicine; Dr. Ho Guangren, Guangren Diabetes Research Center; Dr. Wang Faming, Liaoning Chinese Traditional Medicine Institute; and Dr. Feng Pu as our advisor and mentor.

Over the last ten years we have benefited from the support of Dr. Tom Grade and Dr. Klee Bethel of Baywood Pain Management; Dr. Ronald Sampson; Dr. Jon Porman, Chiropractic Sports and Family Clinic; Dr. Caron Petersen, Health Oasis and Anti-Aging Institute; Dr. Robert Tully; Dr. Farra Swan; Dr. Nick Buratovich; Dr. Greg Curtis; Dr. Andy and Patty Pivonka of Pivonka Family Chiropractic; and Dr. Jeffrey Mainland.

We give special thanks to the editorial help provided by William Hoffman, Judy Hoffman, and Patricia Spadaro for their contribution to our final completion of the book.

Thanks to our sacred and mystic teachers of Taoism and chi-gong, in China and other parts of the world, for their inspirational teaching, not only for the art, but also for the spirit.

Finally, we appreciate the support from our family members, Justin and Jason, Bao Yiaxian, Wu Shouxin, Wang Xin, and Li Sitian.

PREFACE

Our work is different from any you have read. It is the result of experiment and cultivation on ourselves—our own body, mind, and spirit. As the first to benefit from these studies and this research, we have become, in essence, real human test subjects. What we've done is combine the best that modern science has to offer on longevity with methods proven valid over thousands of years of practice.

This work is not another fashionable free lunch on longevity—hot for a couple of years only to be proven ineffective. We don't believe in fashions. What we present is a true journey to vibrant health.

We call our seven protocols *PingLongevity*. The name comes from the Chinese word *ping,* meaning peace, health, and luck. It reflects the tai chi—the perfect blend of yin and yang, with yin in yang, and yang in yin. In people, it means balance and vibrant health.

PingLongevity is a complete way to live younger, more enjoyably, and longer. It consists of seven longevity protocols, eight fundamental herbal formulas, and eight meridian balance tests. The goal is to dramatically increase our life span while looking and feeling decades younger than others in the same age group. It combines thousands of years of Taoism longevity (based on the I-Ching energy cycle, five elements, yin-yang, and Taoist alchemy) and extensive modern anti-aging research. It peels to the very core and explains the things that really make a difference.

Although *PingLongevity* is the result of refining modern and ancient methods, it differs from them too. For example, we recommend eating raw and live food. This is counter to traditional Chinese medicine, which requires eating medium temperature and cooked food. Our program differs from modern medicine too. In many regards, we are controversial in opposing conventional wisdom and fashionable trends. We don't believe in hard exercises. We want to have less wearing and tearing of muscles, tendons, and joints. We don't strictly count vitamins, minerals, proteins, carbohydrates, fats, and fibers. We make sure the body can efficiently absorb and utilize them. We don't believe in feast-and-fast weight control schemes. We want a constant ideal weight. We don't believe that the more hormones (HGH, testosterone, DHEA, etc.), the better. Instead, we look for constant, sustained hormonal balance.

We also don't look at the body as separate organs, tissues, cells, DNA's, and so on. We see the body/mind/spirit as a unified energy system connected to the universe. We agree with the notion that sexual activeness is a sign of vitality, but we differ entirely on the leakage of potent sexual energies as practiced in the modern world. We look for returning to the pre-pubic period as opposed to the accelerated growth to maturity occurring today.

We are realists. We don't wait until everything is "scientifically proven." We consider thousands of years of practice to be more reliable than fly-by-night data advertised in fads. We want to see an impact on our current life rather than waiting many years for advancements in science and technology. We like data-driven science but are very careful in reading it. It is too easy to draw conclusions based on data, which can be only as accurate as you see it. Blind men touching different parts of an elephant will describe the elephant in different ways.

We look for the fundamentals. For example, it is conventional wisdom to increase HGH and testosterone levels as well as metabolic rate. Instead, we seek an efficient body mechanism that would normally keep these at a low level, with an output much more effective than usual. Therefore, the body keeps itself vital for a much longer time.

The method presented here represents our continued research and development of the fundamental longevity method at PingClinic, LLC, and associated doctors, herbalists, and anti-aging research institutions in China.

Ping Wu, M.D.
Taichi Tzu, Ph.D.

CHAPTER 1

HOW OLD ARE WE?

"Ping," asked Frank, on a visit to PingClinic. "I am 45 years old. Since I turned 35, I have been feeling older every year. I don't know how to stop it. I am afraid of getting old."

I had known Frank for more than five years. He is a successful corporate executive, a perfectionist not only in business but also about his health. He was actually an expert in many health-related topics due to an interest in beating the odds of aging. I knew he was in good health and good shape compared to the usual standard.

"I don't think you are in bad shape," I said.

"I just did a biomarker test from an anti-aging doctor," Frank replied. "He told me I am functionally ten years older than my biological age. He said I need to use growth hormones."

"How did you do in the categories he tested?"

"Not well in what is called the forced vital capacity test. The doctor explained that it measures lung function, the amount of air that can be inhaled and exhaled rapidly in one very deep breath. Although I'm 45, I scored a functional age of 60-plus. I also did poorly in a growth hormone test, IGF-1, again about that of a 60-year-old. I thought I was healthier than most people my age. But now I am depressed."

"How was your lung function when you were young? "

"I don't know. I was a 100-meter medallist in high school and college. But I wasn't good at longer ranges, such as 800 meters or 1500 meters. I got tired and out of breath easily."

"So your lung capacity wasn't that high when you were young. Most probably the same test then would have given similar results.

"You think so?"

"Yes, each one of us is different. We were born to be strong in certain areas and weak in others. This does not mean that we were born to be functionally old. Tests use statistical averages. For example, if your test results fall into a range among average Americans in your age group, you are considered normal medically. You may have a low blood pressure of 90/65 compared with your age group, but if you have been at this level all your life and you are healthy, you are fine. You must compare yourself today with your own historical test results. Look for the trend. If the trend takes a downturn at a rate faster than the average, you are aging faster. Doctors can only conclude that you are somewhat within or out of the normal range. But telling your functional age is another matter. I think you may find yourself in the normal functional age for the vital capacity test if you compare the results to your own history of youth."

"What about the tests I did well in?"

"What was your BMI, the body-mass index?"

"About 22. For six feet, 190 pounds, it's perfect, according to the Centers for Disease Control and Prevention standard. I am proud of myself. You know, 61% of Americans are considered overweight."

"Remember what I said: compare yourself with yourself, not with the average. What was your weight at age 20?" I wanted to drive the concept home so Frank could get a correct perception of his health.

"I was about 155 pounds," he said. He thought it over. "You think maybe I am a little overweight compared to my own standard? True, I'm okay compared with the average. But since I was thinner than average genetically, I need to be thinner than the average BMI."

"Exactly. A person's ideal weight is when he is at peak energy, around 18 to 22 years old. As we age, we tend to put on additional weight unnecessarily. We burn our engine not for useful work but to make useless fat. Since the engine can only run a certain number of miles, we accelerate aging unnecessarily. Ideally, if you want to keep your functional youth, maintain your ideal weight throughout life."

I hoped the concept was clear. The biomarkers can only be compared with one's own historical trend.

"What is the most important measurement of youthfulness?" Frank dug deeper and deeper.

"Good question." I took a breath, preparing for a little lecture. "There is a popular biomarker test called the H-Scan Computerized Biological Age Test System. It is based on a few carefully selected standardized biomarkers of aging: reaction time, visual accommodation, forced vital capacity, vibrotactile sensitivity, highest audible pitch, memory recall, alternate button tapping time, muscle movement time, decision reaction time, and decision movement time. You use a specialized computer to answer questions. After about 45 minutes, your biological age is estimated as compared to the statistics of the general population. This type of system should only be used to monitor your own trend, rather than to compare to the standard, as I told you earlier.

"Our approach is different. We don't believe functional age can be accurately estimated. Few of us tracked our biomarkers when we were 20 years old, so there is little to compare against. After all, the purpose is to understand if we are changing rapidly, and to figure out ways to stop or reverse the changes. Therefore, we think testing is for identification of issues and trends, rather than estimating the ages.

"There are a few important things you should track —not to just test once a year but to monitor your own historical trend. First, your metabolic rate. It is related to how fast we live our lives. If you are healthy, the lower the pulse rate (optimally in the low 60's) and the body temperature (1-2 degrees less than the usual 98), the better. The other factor on metabolic rate is how fast we consume food. Increasing body weight is an unhealthy increase of consumption. It is not needed by the body. Always keep your body weight at where it was when you were 18 to 22 years old.

"You should keep your blood healthy—sparkling clean and fluid. This means keeping a low level of blood fat, usually measured by cholesterol (optimally in the low 100's), blood sugar (optimally in the 70's), blood pressure (less than 110), and toxins. Toxins arise from undesirable lifestyles, such as smoking, drinking, eating junk food, and taking in polluted air and water. Clean and fluid blood can, without straining the heart pump, easily flow into every little vein of the body, bringing in nutrients and oxygen and taking away waste products. This helps all parts of your body function well. On the other hand, if your blood fat content is high, sugar is high, and pressure is high and your blood is full of toxins from the environment and food as well as stress, the blood becomes very dense. It's like trying to make honey flow through a thin straw. As a result, the blood won't reach the remote, vital parts of the body easily.

"Next, you should make sure your energy is sufficient. I am not only talking about feeling full of energy but about subtle energy, which flows through your body's energy channels. In Chinese traditional medicine, this subtle energy is called chi, and the channels are called meridians. There is no modern equipment or technology that can yet adequately measure this subtle energy.

Some new equipment measures people's energy in terms of the color spectrum but may not show the higher energies.

"Chi sustains life. Chi must be balanced through all meridians. We can tell how strong your chi is and how balanced you are through reading your vital signs. The body's major energy systems are linked to the openings and surfaces of the body. For example, the liver energy system is responsible for making and storing blood as well as synthesizing fuel for the body. The energy of the liver is reflected in the eyes. Red, unclear eyes indicate a possible blockage of liver energy through its meridian. By reading your vital signs through your face, eye, ear, lip, tongue, and other physiological feelings and phenomena throughout the body, we can have a pretty good idea about your energy balance and vitality. I'll teach you our vital sign test and balancing herbal formulas later.

"If you can maintain your ideal body weight, keep your blood vibrant and fluid, and have high energy balance, the next step is to check your sexual vitality. Sexual energy is not just for sex. It determines whether we have high energy and high vital essence in our body. Both energy and essence are required to maintain a youthful life. Compared to yourself at age 20, are you maintaining the same sexual desire, potency, high erection angles, and sufficient semen? Frequent sexual activities also stimulate your hormonal systems, affecting your growth hormone and testosterone levels. A healthy level of these hormones results in lean muscle, fast cell repair, and sexual potency.

"The next major indicator is mind and spirituality. When you are young, say age 15, you are relatively naïve. Your mind is not complicated. Your desires and cravings are simple. You are not into power, money, sex, food, or fame. Thus your stress is low. Stress is a main accelerator of aging. Therefore, you need to maintain no greater stress level than when you were basically a kid, no matter what happens around you, such as legal problems, power struggles, divorce, wealth, fame, or work.

"Lastly, there are a few additional tests usually performed by anti-aging doctors: hormone test, forced vital capacity, auto-antibodies, static balance, and skin elasticity. It is important to make sure you only compare with yourself, not the average population. Look at the rate of deterioration over time and keep it as slow as possible throughout your life."

"I am overwhelmed," Frank said, "about how fast these things decline."

I paused, then launched into a recitation of facts that Frank, and so many others, need to know:

- Weight increases to about age 55, then begins to fall.
- The drop in weight between 55 and 75 is due mostly to loss of lean tissue, muscle mass, water, and bone.

I stopped for a moment. "What's important to you," I said to Frank, "is what happens between age 20 and 60":

- The percentage of overweight people doubles from 20% to more than 40%, according to 1991 government statistics. The amount of fat doubles.
- Blood fat content increases. LDL, the bad cholesterol, and triglycerides, a fat in blood, increases by about 40%.
- The blood sugar level surges. Diabetes increases by about ninefold, from 1.5% of all Americans at age 20 to 13% by age 60.
- Cardiovascular system function declines. The VO2max, maximum consumption rate of oxygen during strenuous exercises such as a treadmill, declines about 25%, thus lessening ability to play intense sports.

- Hormone level decreases dramatically. DHEA decreases by about 65%, HGH (the growth hormone) by about 60%, and testosterone by 40%.
- Sexual vitality reduces significantly. Frequency of sexual orgasms reduces by about 65% from about 104 times a year to 35 times. Erection angle for men declines from 20 degrees to –25 degrees.
- Bone density, measured in the hip, decreases by about 20%, increasing the chance of fractures.
- Forced vital capacity declines about 40%.
- Hearing a higher pitched sound (8000 frequency) requires the sound to be 8 times louder.
- Static balance is tested by standing on a hard floor, with eyes closed, lifting one leg about six inches off the floor. Time before falling over decreases sixfold, from more than 30 seconds to less than 5 seconds.
- Brain function is reduced too. About 35% of people develop Alzheimer's disease by age 75, and 50% develop it by age 85.

"That's very depressing," Frank sighed. "Why do people have to age at all? Wouldn't it be nice if we just stayed young, and died suddenly after 80 years?"

"There are actually living things which do not get old, such as sharks, sea turtles, and whales," I said, continuing my lecturing. "Rockfish, the ones we eat at our dinner table, are usually over 100 years old. Nobody really knows why. There are more than 25 modern and a great many more ancient theories on aging. It's impossible for me to talk about them all. But let me mention a few. One is the Disposable Soma Theory, with a hypothesis that the purpose of our body/life is for procreation only. Thus after procreation, life is destroyed. Evolution has selected the species that maximizes procreation of offspring at the expense of longer life.

"Another theory is based on the Wear-and-Tear hypothesis. Animals get old just like cars do. Elephants die because they wear down their teeth so much that they can no longer eat properly.

"Another theory uses a Rate-of-Living hypothesis. It states that there is a metabolic 'bank' account. People can consume a limited amount of total fuel or calories throughout life. The quicker we consume that total, the faster we die.

"There is also the Oxidative-Stress Theory. You often hear about free radicals and anti-oxidants in dietary supplement ads. This theory says that as we metabolize glucose as fuel, the free radicals, or oxidant byproduct, combines with proteins, etc., to form damaged cells. As time goes by, these damaged cells accumulate, just as rust inside a car engine accumulates over time. Since our body burns fuel (glucose) with the help of oxygen breathed in through the lung and carried by blood, it has a mechanism similar to an automobile engine burning gasoline with the help of air (or oxygen). No body system or car engine is 100% efficient, so byproducts are created over time. The biggest byproduct is oxides, which rust the inner parts of a car's engine. They also 'rust' the cells of our body."

"There seems no easy way out," said Frank. "We have to get old and die. But how can I prolong youthful life?"

"Yes. We all get old and die. But we can double our life span. If the average life expectancy is 75 years, we can live over 150 years, and extend our young life from 45 to 75 or older!"

"Should I take growth hormones and the anti-aging plan my doctor suggested? He really believes his anti-aging plan with growth hormone replacement therapy and herbal supplements is the fountain of youth."

"Do the people look dramatically younger than normal by taking the plan?"

"No. Many visitors to the office were bald, look old, and are overweight. Even the doctor himself seems to have low energy and keeps drinking coffee. I was wondering how I could believe someone who preaches a wonder anti-aging plan which cannot save his own fountain of youth?"

"The problem with most drugs is that they function via only one specific mechanism. By affecting just one metabolic pathway, biochemical and subtle energy imbalances can develop in the body that often result in the dangerous side effects characteristic of prescription drugs. For example, drugs that inhibit the cyclooxyenase-2 enzyme have shown efficacy in alleviating inflammation and pain caused by arthritis. However, a study published in the August 2000 issue of the *Journal of Immunology* identifies a potential long-term problem that could lead to cartilage and other tissue degeneration if these drugs are taken over an extended period. "Another example is estrogen used in hormone replacement therapy. Estrogen is being considered for listing in the next federal Report on Carcinogens. It's been pretty well accepted for a number of years that the hormonal effects of estrogen have led to endometrial cancer in women. Millions of people have tried wonder drugs—Rezulin for diabetes, silicone breast implant, Viagra, to name just a few—only to find significant side effects.

"About anti-aging methods. There are more than 25 modern theories of aging and a great number of doctors offering different ways of anti-aging. Many are a correct method but not a complete method. It is similar to the blind attempting to describe an elephant by touching only one of its parts. Thus they came up with the trunk method, the tusk method, the ear method, the tail method, the leg method, and so on. The fact is that a million things can be proven beneficial to health in one aspect or another. There are millions of different herbs, fruits, and vegetables in nature which can be proven to have some health benefit, such as reduce the risk of cancer. But can we take them all? Is the effect too little to be really practical?"

Frank asked, "Are you talking about a perfect world? How can I achieve ideal weight, vibrant fluid blood, high energy, highly developed mind and spirituality, great sexual vitality…all you have mentioned? I've done studies of anti-aging methods. You are talking about something very different."

Frank tried to hurry me to the bottom line. Like most baby boomers, Frank enjoys life so much and has noticed that it passes very quickly. He has felt the test of time—the imprints on his own reduced vitality—and is attempting in vain to stop it. Now he is fighting for his own survival.

"If you are as determined as you sound, I'll teach you the method of *PingLongevity*. It is a complete way to live younger, more enjoyably, and longer. The goal is to live a life 10 to 50 years younger than most people in the same age group. It combines thousands of years of Taoism longevity (based on the I-Ching energy cycle, the five elements theory, the yin-yang principle, and Taoist alchemy) plus extensive modern anti-aging research to really make a difference. It's never too late. Even if you have already been suffering from degenerative diseases of older age, you can reverse it. It's never too early either. Aging starts at puberty. You can preserve energy and stop aging now."

"I'd like to start right now," Frank said, eagerly.

CHAPTER 2

THE UNIVERSAL LAWS OF ENERGY AND LIFE

Deep into the foggy little mountain path, we saw a small figure in front of us climbing the steep rocky slope, framed against a background of beautiful lush greens. There was a refreshing, energizing breeze. It was our second day at the mystic and sacred Ching Cheng Mountain, the birthplace of Taoism in Shezhuan Province, on our annual trip to China seeking the truth about longevity. A charming lady who looked to be in her 60's was taking a rest in front of us. "Hello, my friends," she said.

Still catching our breath, we answered, "Hello. Are you from around here, and what are you doing so deep in the mountain?"

Opening a huge bag, she explained, "Yes. I live down at the foot of the mountain. I am collecting herbs. This one is to increase vitality. This increases chi. The one over here is to channel the meridians."

"Do people here all take these herbs? Do they live long?"

"We all take herbs. I am 92 years old."

We were shocked. "Really, are you 92? What is the secret to being so agile and healthy at your age?"

"Well, it is not unusual for us to live to this age. We have quite a few who are much older," she said matter of factly.

"May I take a picture with you? I am really impressed."

Considering all we have discovered during our annual trips to China seeking out the learned ones, I thought how wonderful it would be if millions of people could know even half of these secrets of vibrant health.

Ping's Diary

Five thousand years ago, the Taoist sages of China formulated the understanding of the laws of the universe, the Oracle of Changes (I Ching), and the complex acupuncture meridians as the paths of energy through the human body.

It is remarkable that today modern science and technology have confirmed the validity of these ancient perceptions of the world and the human body. It has been found that the meridians of the ancients correspond to paths in the body with low electrical resistance, even though the meridians are not found in modern physiology to correspond to any physical structures, i.e., blood vessels, lymph nodes, or nerves.

More amazing, it has also been found (around 1969 independently by Dr. Gunther Stent, Dr. Martin Schonberger, Dr. Marie-Louise von Franz, and others) that the 64 I Ching code is identical to the genetic code of DNA, which describes the entire living world and was discovered less than fifty years ago.

How could these ancients be right on the mark? How were they able to perceive truths that even now modern men struggle to measure and comprehend? Quite a feat for a prehistoric people who had no written language, no science, no technological instruments, no mathematics. They recorded numbers by tying knots on a blade of grass.

The answer, most likely, is that the ancients were a pure and simple people, their observations not obstructed by the hundreds of distractions we have today. They studied existence as it is—a skill now lost, perhaps through evolution. They perceived nature through a clear lens. Stories talk about ancient herbalists discovering many of the precious herbs. It is said that while climbing high into the mountains, they would pass by a new plant and feel a sensation through different body parts. This gave them an understanding of the healing effect of herbs on specific parts of the body.

The ancient laws, combined with modern research and scientific methodology, are the foundations of this book. We're talking here about laws that dictate how long we live and how we age. Now bolstered by modern science, these laws have been proven for thousands of years in real life. Since they are critical to our state of being, health, and longevity, it is vital to understand and implement them.

Each of us has a limited life span. Life, in fact, is short. Our peak energy years, which begin at puberty, number about fifteen. Our goal is to increase the overall life span, while improving its quality and vitality. The idea is to live longer and healthier.

Taoist alchemy started with the first Chinese king, Huang Di (the Yellow Emperor), about 5,000 years ago. Unlike a religion where people say prayers to get blessings, Taoist alchemy believes in self-cultivation and refinement. It is a science set out to explain the laws of the universe and life. It is about the macrocosm of the universe, and the microcosm of humans. It observes nature to understand human beings and observes human beings to understand the universe. In development and verification over several thousands of years, Taoist alchemy became the science and the art of self-refinement of spiritual (original nature) and physical (vital life-force) lives. Its ultimate goal is to combine life with the Tao, or the ultimate universal chi (energy), to achieve longevity. It believes that our limited life force has all it takes to refine ourselves into immortality and grand happiness, regardless of fate. It is up to us to achieve it.

Taoist alchemy believes in the combined training of both spirit and physical life. It appears to be between religion (pure spiritual) and science (pure material). It requires that body, mind, and spirit be one and that the macrocosm of the universe and the microcosm of the human be one. It is through this combination that man, with very limited life, can achieve immortality by communicating with the infinite energy of the universe. According to the old Taoist saying, "Universe has limited life span, my spirit energy can last forever!"

THE LAW OF ENERGY

The ancient Chinese believed that the universe is filled with energy, that energy is everything. Indeed, much of this has been proven: electromagnetic fields, light beams, and gravity fields have all been measured. But the ancients, right in so many things, believed in a continuum of energies, from the lowest level (unstable, impure, mortal, coarse, of the lower spectrum) to the highest level (subtle, immortal, infinite, pure, absolute, perfect, refined, of the higher spectrum).

Perfect energy is called the Tao or chi, a force flowing within us and filling the universe. It is the energy that created all things. The Tao divides into yin and yang energy. Yin and yang energies give birth to all things, which are themselves the manifestation of these energies. Once things take on physical form, such as mountains, trees, animals, humans, electromagnetic fields, they become mortal. They have limited life energy potential. As the energy is expended, things are dissolved back into the universe (for example, living things die and mountains ultimately disappear through eruption of volcanoes). Most important to our understanding of life is that *mortality rate or life span depends on the quality of the energy in its position between the spectrum of lowest to highest energies and the rate of energy expenditure.* The higher the quality of the energy and the slower the consumption rate, the longer the thing stays stable.

Albert Einstein's theory of relativity holds that all energy and matter are interchangeable. It depends on the speed at which matter is moving or vibrating. As the speed approaches that of light, the energy increases towards infinity, and matter becomes mass-less. This is described in Einstein's celebrated mass-energy formula:

$$E = M \frac{c^2}{\sqrt{1 - (v/c)^2}}$$

where E stands for energy, M for mass, c for the speed of light, and v for the vibrational speed of the mass.

This is in agreement with the ancients in that the universe is filled with energies. Energies have their associated speed. At lower speeds, energies are condensed into physical existence. As the speed increases, energies become subtle, formless, and mass-less. In living things, the higher the vibration of energy, the longer and more stable its life.

Physicists use the term *entropy* to describe the disorganization of things or the randomness of a system. The greater the degree of disorder, the higher the entropy. In thermodynamics, a formula $S = H - G$ is used to describe the relationship among entropy S, heat H, and energy potential available for useful work G in a closed thermodynamic system. Thus, the less the energy potential G, the higher is the entropy S (the tendency toward disorganization). The higher the energy consumed, represented by heat H, the higher is the entropy. Thermodynamics holds that all closed systems (approximately applied to humans, not entirely a closed system) have positive entropy, which always increases as time goes by, so the system ultimately becomes more and more disorganized until it destroys itself and dies. This agrees very much with the ancient Chinese view of the universe that lower energy forms are mortal and instable.

Until recently, energy vibrating at faster than the speed of light was considered impossible. However, physicists have now hypothesized the possibility of a negative space/time. As noted in Einstein's formula, when v is larger than c, energy E becomes an imaginary number, thus the name negative space/time. In such a space/time, energy vibrating faster than the speed of light would cause living systems to possess negative entropy (sometimes called extropy), increasing order and organization as time goes by, and actually enhance the system's ability to live a longer, more stable, and even immortal existence. The higher the vibration of the energies, the more stable they stay. This hypothesis by modern physicists again agrees with the ancients—the higher the energy, the more immortal it is.

THE LAW OF LIFE

The law of life, called the energy cycle of I Ching, states that when there is birth, there must be a death. Birth grows out of death, and death occurs in birth. The universe of transformation is periodic and yin-yang balanced.

I Ching represents yin with a broken line and yang with a solid line. Then I Ching stacks six broken and solid lines into a hexagram representing one state. There are 64 different combinations of the six lines, with broken or solid lines in all six positions.

These 64 hexagrams represent 64 different states of change in the universe. The hexagram grows from bottom to top. Thus, one broken line at the bottom and five solid lines at the top means there is a recent birth of yin into the new state. When the different hexagrams are put in order, they describe a change process or law in the universe, living things, or events going from one state to another. The law of life is shown below.

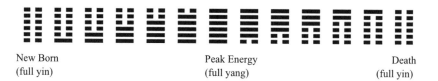

New Born   Peak Energy   Death
(full yin)   (full yang)   (full yin)

Life starts at birth, which is at the full yin state (six yin lines), and reaches its peak energy at full yang state (six yang lines), with a gradual increase of yang from the bottom up, representing the increase of energy. After the peak energy state, life begins a gradual slide. This downhill process is represented by an increase of yin (broken lines) from the bottom up until full yin is reached, when death returns to birth and a cycle ends.

As you can see, if you add the hexagrams together, it is yin-yang balanced (the number of yin and yang are equal, and the periodical life process itself is yin and yang balanced).

"Peak energy" in people occurs at puberty when male and female become capable of reproduction, with the first leakage of semen (male) and blood in menstrual period (female). Today the physiological peak is reached earlier than in the past, since people "mature" faster in our food-stuffed, sex-driven, materialistic society. Growth has been accelerated in the race to reach maturity.

Longevity not only depends on how fast one reaches the peak energy state, but it also depends on the quality (vibrational speed) of one's energy and how fast energy is consumed.

All humans possess three treasures: spirit, chi, and essence. They are energies in three different manifestations with different vibrational speeds, spirit being the highest and essence the lowest. And all humans have pure and impure energy components; the purer, the longer they live. Conversely, the more impure, the shorter they live. The faster they consume the limited energy potential, the quicker the rate toward death.

At conception, pure spirit energy enters to combine with the vital essence of the parents (the sperm of the father and egg of the mother) as well as the mother's nursing chi to form the seed of new life. This is the basic beginning of life—the prenatal energy. Inside the womb, yin (in the form of essence) and yang (in the form of spirit) are in perfect union.

At birth, yin and yang separate and the I Ching life cycle begins. Spirit (subconscious mind) and mind (conscious mind) goes upwards to be housed in the brain and the heart, and essence goes down to be stored in the kidneys. Postnatal essence builds up through the digestion of nutrients from food. Together, the spirit energy and the essence sustain the life-force, the chi. Life is supported by chi; strong spirit and essence support strong chi, which in turn supports life. Throughout life, spirit leaks upwards through emotions, while essence leaks downward in the form of enzymes, semen, blood, eggs, body fluids, and through the metabolism processes. As vital essence and spirit energies are depleted, chi is gradually weakened. Since chi cannot sustain life, so life ends.

Prior to puberty, children are naïve and relatively mindless. They usually do not relate to things like fame, wealth, success, social standards, and stress. Therefore, spiritual energy is largely preserved. Leakage of semen and blood (through menstrual period) has not begun. Essence is also preserved. Therefore, the life-force, or chi energy, is increasing and will peak at puberty.

Clearly, if puberty can be delayed, so too will the aging process. We can stay younger longer. But, instead of delaying the aging process, modern lifestyles have accelerated it. Children grow up faster, mature faster, are physically larger, and enter puberty earlier.

Much of this is caused by processed food and the methods used to raise animals, e.g., growing chicken in a caged environment, despite the fact that uncaged, "wild" chicken tastes better and is more nutritious. In the same vein, wild fruits and vegetables are healthier for humans, yet we stuff ourselves with chemical and hormone-filled food. We are shortening our healthy lives span.

After puberty, on the spiritual level, stress begins to accumulate. We start to understand power, social status, fame, money, politics, sexual attraction, and the pressures of work. The spirit becomes overpowered by modern realities, and spirit energy decreases as these take their toll. As spirit energy diminishes, chi is weakened and so too is life.

Civilization and modernization accelerate the process, and many of us are overwhelmed by this information age: the Internet, television, newspapers, and ads. It seems everyone in the world wants to sell us something.

This becomes clear to people lucky enough to visit a primitive village in a remote place. The people there spend a lot of time sitting around and doing nothing. They make a living—growing crops, picking fruit, making clothing—but aren't distracted by the sirens of modernity. Mainly they seem to enjoy themselves and have fun.

After puberty, our essence begins to slide downhill. Nutrition helps slow the decline, but processed foods dilute the benefits. The release of semen (in sex) and blood (from menstruation) weakens the crucial reserve of essence. The other most critical consumers of essence are enzymes, of which we have a limited supply.

You may ask, "Isn't it true that life expectancy has increased from 50 years at the turn of the 1900's to around 76 years by the end of the century? Isn't that a help instead of harm to health and life span?" Yes. It is true that life expectancy has increased, but that is mainly attributable to the invention of antibiotics and the corresponding reduction in communicable infectious diseases as well as the increased availability of nutrition, the increase of birth survival rate, and the medical advancement of replacing malfunctioning body parts (blocked veins, heart valves, hip joints, liver, blood, etc.). There has been, on the other hand, a dramatic increase of degenerative diseases such as diabetes, osteoporosis, cancer, AIDS, obesity—a true indicator of internal health.

How fast will we age? What is the most important factor that determines the rate of aging? What can we do to add significant, healthful, productive years to our lives? This book answers these vital questions.

In a nutshell, the rate of aging depends on the quality of our energies and how fast spirit and essence are depleted. It is said that longevity is 60% dependent on the genes and 40% on the environment (the style of living). This modern claim is consistent with the Taoist's perception of quality of energy and rate of living. Taoist alchemy together with modern sciences can change both, not through future genetic therapies but rather through today's cultivation of yourself, starting right now with yourself. You'll understand as you read on.

Both the ancient Chinese masters and modern scientists estimate that humans have a maximum life span of 100 to 120 years. In fact, if we could cure all heart diseases and all cancer and eliminate all the causes of death written on death certificates today so that all people die only from "natural causes," almost everyone would live to be about 100 years old according to statistics. Can we have an effective program to help people live to their maximum life span of around 100 to 120? Can we dramatically increase this maximum limit to over 200? The answers are both yes. Do you want to live that long?

What matters is how healthy your life is. An individual may quite honestly say that longevity is not his goal; what matters is the quality of life.   With this there can be no disagreement. When we extend our healthy life span, we also extend our younger life span. In order to live 150 healthy years, we must have the physical and mental health of the traditional middle age of a 45-year-old when in fact we are in our 70's. Thus, in effect, we must extend our young and middle ages. Extending life span or longevity also means we have to delay all age-related degenerative diseases, such as cancer, heart problems, and osteoporosis. This is also consistent with the goal of quality of life.

THE *PINGLONGEVITY* PROTOCOLS

The maximum life span, living happily and in good health, can often be achieved if spirit and essence energy are maximally preserved, so that the life-sustaining chi is maintained. It was called "happily lived maximum" in ancient times, referring to those who lived more than one hundred years in good health.

As will be demonstrated, people are capable of living much longer than 120 years and doing it in a completely productive manner.

Increasing life span, and maximum life span, requires our making some fundamental changes: becoming a being with a higher vibrating energy. As discussed earlier, the stability (or immortality) of a form depends on both the rate of energy consumption and the quality of the energy, i.e., its frequency of vibration. The more the energy is taking physical forms, the less its vibrating frequency. The physical form disappears as the speed goes equal or beyond that of light, as we have seen earlier in Einstein's formula. Spirit energy is the highest and most refined in our human energy spectrum; vital essence such as blood, semen, enzyme, and body fluids are lower and coarser energies. They both sustain chi to support the existence of life. At death, our essence is drained, and spirit energy is weakened through lifelong consumption. Chi is insufficient to sustain life. Thus, our physical body dies and our spirit energy reunites with the universe.

If we can daily preserve and lower the expenditure of our spirit and essence energy, we can sustain a strong chi longer and achieve longevity towards the human maximum limit. Furthermore, if we can use our vital essence energy as raw materials, and refine it into higher chi and spirit energy, we can challenge the maximum limit and move towards immortality—an energy so refined that it lasts forever.

How do we preserve and refine our energies? We need to prevent vital essence, such as blood, semen, enzymes, and body fluids, from unnecessary expenditure. We need to open and balance our energy meridians and centers in order not to accumulate illness (caused by imbalance and blockage) and to be in touch with the infinite cosmic energy source of the universe. We need to calm our spirit from all emotional stress to preserve our spirit energy. We need to transmute the essence energy into higher chi and spirit energy.

Our program consists of seven protocols, based on the laws of the energy universe, the law of living, and several breathtaking modern scientific advances in the field of longevity.

The protocols can be divided into three areas: Area 1 deals with the conservation of vital essence; Area 2 with the energy plane, the opening and balancing of meridians and energy centers; and Area 3 with spiritual energy preservation and refinement.

All three areas apply ancient and modern research methodology to achieve maximum benefits.

The ancients taught that spiritual healing is superior to other methods, that energy healing is next, that food healing is excellent, that herbal healing is good, and that chemical and/or surgi-cal healing should be sought only as a last resort. Though discuss-ing all, this book will focus mainly on spiritual, energy, and food healing.

We'd like to acknowledge that many of us will not adhere to all seven protocols or not follow them to the letter. Life is a process of tradeoffs. A diabetes patient, for example, may choose to ingest sugar, despite the risk, because he rationalizes either that it may not hurt—just this once—or that life itself is not tolerable if a craving this strong isn't satisfied.

A major reason this program has proved successful is that exercising serious restraints is not required. No one is expected to abandon the enjoyment of things he really enjoys.

Taoism is natural. It teaches that people should follow their internal nature. It seeks to convert negative forces in society, forces opposed to longevity, into something positive. Thus, there is no need to force yourself to do anything. Reducing the intake of calories will no doubt reduce the rate of living, thus extending life. Avoiding too much starchy, processed, and cooked food will surely reduce the expenditure of the very precious enzymes—part of vital essence. But we are not advocating hunger or eating things you don't enjoy.

On the contrary, our protocols have ways to keep you full with low calorie intake and provide flexibility for meals you like. You should feel dramatically energized through the food protocols because your body will expend less energy burning calories to make fat and will conserve more enzymes for growth and repair rather than digestion.

PingLongevity, the complete way of life for a young, healthy, and long-lasting body and spirit, features three levels of development and can benefit virtually everyone, regardless of his/her ability to link with nature and spirituality. Everyone can apply it at the physical level; some can apply it to the energy level;

and, although difficult, some can reach the spiritual plane. What-
ever goal you achieve, the benefits will be enormous.

LET'S GET BACK TO NATURE

Advances in civilization have no doubt increased our survival rate. Humans learned to build shelters to protect against at-
tacks by wild animals and severe weather. Our ancestors invented
farming to stave off hunger; antibiotics to guard against contagious
diseases; and medical procedures, including blood transfusions,
hormone replacement, and organ transplants, to repair the body. In
the meantime, these very advancements have taken us step-by-step
away from nature.

There have been serious consequences.

The invention of fire led to the cooking of food, depriving
people of natural energy components: live energy, food enzymes,
etc.

The invention of farming meant humans could consume
food not naturally intended for them, such as rice and flour. In their
original form, such foods have enzyme inhibitors and are indi-
gestible in a human system, but in a cooked form they are highly
starchy and enzyme-less.

The invention of the mass storing and processing of food
deprived it of whole nutrition, further de-energized the food, and
made it highly insulin sensitive, resulting in increased obesity and
type II diabetes. What we have is an overweight generation with
numerous degenerative diseases that were unknown before.

But the list goes on. Synthesized chemicals are added to
food during processing, chemical fertilizers are introduced into our
over-farmed soils, and hormones and antibiotics are fed to farm-
grown animals. These in turn are transferred into the human body,

generating accelerated growth. As mentioned, people grow faster and age faster.

Finally, humans have become the busiest species on the planet. We can learn from animals, including cats and dogs, which spend most of their time relaxing, their spirits relatively pure. The same is true of certain primitive tribes, people not burdened by bewildering rules, regulations, laws, and policies— in other words, unnatural stresses. They don't worry about having to fight for status, fame, or money. They are not regularly bombarded with sexually saturated inducements. All these things create stress, and stress is a killer.

We have learned, through the creation of nuclear weapons, how to mass self-destruct. Perhaps just as deadly, poisonous substances have been leaked into our land, air, and water. How do we protect ourselves until safer policies prevail?

We are transitioning into a totally wireless society: cellular phones, wireless home networking, wireless Internet, wireless control of home appliances, cars with GPS (Global Positioning Systems). We will be living in the middle of waves.

We are even beginning to genetically alter ourselves and the surroundings. Our very nature, and those of plants and animals, are being changed in a radical way.

This book is not intended to be alarmist. Rather, its purpose is to help people live longer, healthier, more satisfying lives in a climate not designed for any of this.

Civilization has enhanced our survival rate, but it also has denatured us. Showing how to combat this denaturization is the vital message of this book.

CHAPTER 3

FIRST PROTOCOL:
EAT LIVE ENERGY FOOD

"Ping," said Susan, one of my friends, at lunch with me and my friend Dr. Russ, "I'm really frustrated about my health. I am overweight and now have diabetes. I tried to lose weight with Fen-Phen, Meridia, Xenical. Now they say these drugs are dangerous. I hired personal trainers, worked out, even fasted. But nothing seems to help."

"Well," Doctor Russ interrupted, "there is no free lunch. People want to take a pill and make up for all their sins. Remember silicon breast implants, estrogen and progesterone hormone replacement? Millions who used them are now suffering side effects. The medical community still hasn't solved the problem of obesity."

He took a long swallow of iced tea and continued: "I just read a report by the National Academy of Sciences, which said insufficient evidence exists to support claims that taking megadoses of dietary antioxidants, such as selenium and vitamins C and E, or carotenoids, including beta-carotine, can prevent chronic diseases."

"And who knows," Susan added, "what the new trends—HGH, sex steroids, DHEA, Viagra, Metabolife, cosmetic surgery—will produce?" She seemed more desperate and confused.

"I agree with Dr. Russ," I said. "There is really no free lunch. Many modern medical solutions can band-aid our lives back together. Heart valve replacement, bypass surgery, hip joint replacement, liposuction, growth hormone replacement all help us stay alive. We must ask ourselves, what are the fundamental causes of these conditions? Band-aids only help us temporarily. The life machine is too complicated to just patch up. We need to take the long road to stay young and have vibrant health."

"Ping," Susan said, "I really agree with you. But after so many false starts, is it too late for me? I have already passed half of my life in such bad shape."

"No. Absolutely not. We have patients who came to us in their seventies. Let's begin your PingLongevity program tomorrow."

The prospect that our longevity program may help millions of people improve their health gets me really excited.

Ping's Diary

Living things are constantly going through chemical processes such as burning energy, storing energy, synthesizing protein, breaking down food, expelling toxins, making new cells, and repairing damaged DNA. They have the machinery needed to liberate and store chemical energy from foods and to create complex molecules from simpler ones for the building of new structures. These processes collectively are called metabolism and involve the transformation by enzyme-catalyzed reactions of both matter and energy.

Enzymes, a kind of protein, are the chemical agents necessary for every chemical reaction to take place. Without enzymes, all functions come to a stop. There is no energy production, no muscle contraction, no breathing, no digestion. According to the ancient law of living, every living thing has a fixed energy potential. Similarly, modern scientists believe there is a limit to our total enzyme potential. During our lifetime, they say, we are capable of producing only a certain amount of enzymes. When there are insufficient enzymes in the body, many critical chemical reactions, such as cell repair, don't occur efficiently or don't occur at all. As a result, the body becomes diseased and aging is accelerated. The faster we produce and use up enzymes, the faster we age.

Thus, metabolism is the sum of all life processes, and enzymes are the agents of all metabolism. Without enzymes, we simply die. A key to vibrant health and long life is to preserve our body's limited number of enzymes as long as possible. One way to do this is to eat natural food that has its own enzymes so that we don't have to expend our own supply of enzymes to digest what we eat.

Digestive enzymes help break down food into usable nutrients and fuels. They are found in saliva, pancreas secretion, and stomach and small intestine digestive fluids. Today it is easy to waste a large amount of our total enzyme potential on producing digestive enzymes because the food we consume has so little enzyme content of its own. By depending on the enzymes already in our food, it is possible to save up to 50% of our body's digestive enzymes.

To understand how we expend our precious enzyme potential, we must first understand nature's laws of food and how we can work with those laws.

NATURE'S FIRST LAW OF FOOD

We eat living things (plants and animals) and take in air (oxygen) to absorb the necessary fuel (calories) and nutrients for sustaining life. By nature's design, every living thing has its own specialized chemicals, called food enzymes, to decompose itself at the proper temperature and moisture levels. Food enzymes are destroyed at a temperature above 110°F and are usually most effective at around 98°F with the right moisture condition. True, 110°F is below the generally recommended temperature for cooking food. On the other hand, a moist 98°F equals conditions in the human stomach, where food is pre-digested.

Therefore, *every living thing contains the exact food enzyme to decompose itself under optimal conditions—and these conditions are identical to the natural environment of the human digestive tract. We are in tune with this law of food when we eat food in a state where its enzymes are alive.*

Some foods are supposed to be eaten raw and fresh because that is when they are enzyme rich. Another way to keep a food's natural enzyme alive is to prepare it pickled, sprouted, low-temperature smoked or naturally dried.

Grains and seeds are a special type of living food. Nature has made them for storage. Therefore, a much longer time is needed, under the right temperature and moisture condition, for their enzymes to take effect. This is because they contain a substance called an enzyme inhibitor, which keeps the enzymes from being effective in the food's raw state.

Because their food enzymes are inhibited, raw grains and seeds are difficult for us to digest. For us to break down the enzymes in raw foods, our bodies need to produce additional digestive enzymes. After wild food became less available, early man learned to farm and cook grains. But the cooking process destroys the food's enzymes.

The best way for us to unlock the enzyme inhibitors in grains and seeds and still preserve their natural enzymes is to eat grains and seeds in a sprouted or fermented state. This is how chickens, birds, and squirrels eat them. A chicken, for example, has a craw, a sort of pre-stomach, which stores grains for days and causes it to ferment before real digestion. Squirrels bury seeds until they sprout. Then they dig out the seed and eat the tender sprout. In both cases, living food is eaten in its natural state and digestion depends on natural enzymes—the food's own decomposing chemicals.

Another good way to eat grains and seeds is when they are very young. Very young corn, for example, can be eaten raw because it is so soft and milky inside.

Unfortunately, developed nations with modern technologies have many new inventions that destroy the natural benefit of food enzymes. For example, in order to mass produce, store, and market food products, all sorts of bacteria must be killed—under the same conditions that kill food enzymes. As a result of the desire to store food for long amounts of time, the food industry cooks, pasteurizes (milk, fruit juice), and processes (packaged vegetables).

As a consequence of eating foods prepared in this way, more and more people are overweight and are plagued by degenerative diseases. We have developed a body system that adapts to enzyme-less food, a system forced to produce huge amounts of digestive enzymes. Because so much of our enzyme potential is used to produce digestive enzymes, our capability for producing enzymes for other metabolic functions, such as maintaining a strong immune system and cell rebuilding, has become deficient. This is why wildlife in their natural habitat do not suffer from degenerative diseases. They usually die only when killed by predators, natural disasters, and contagious diseases caused by deadly epidemics.

Modern man has greatly accelerated the rate of enzyme depletion. It becomes obvious that eating food in its raw state or in a state that keeps food enzymes alive (pickled, sprouted, low-temperature smoked, naturally dried) will dramatically preserve the body's enzyme essence, reduce the rate of aging, and prevent or delay degenerative diseases.

NATURE'S SECOND LAW OF FOOD

According to the universal law of energy, every living thing has a blend of energies of different vibrational frequencies. Our food, therefore, has a physical frequency as well as a higher energy.

Modern science and medicine have only emphasized the need for "nutrition" from the physical constituents of the food because of an inability to understand and measure higher energy. While the physical nutrients are important, they are a lower form of energy compared to the food's higher energy of chi and spirit.

All living things possess the higher energy of chi and spirit, which is attached to the living form. When the physical form dies, the higher energy disperses. When we consume food in its natural state, we can absorb its higher energy. For example, when a living thing, such as an apple, dies, the higher energy leaves its physical form. When we consume food in its natural state, fresh and raw, we also absorb its higher energy, which is incapable of being measured by modern instruments.

NATURE'S THIRD LAW OF FOOD

Living whole foods—including fruits, fish, beans, seeds, and unprocessed meat of different textures and flavors—are digested slowly in the human body because some parts of them are not quickly decomposable. Nature's wild animals have their systems tuned to digesting food slowly over many hours. *Thus, living whole food is meant to be digested slowly, little by little. When we eat foods that are slower to digest, we get more benefit from the food.*

Civilization has made giant steps in refining foods, such as making flours refined from grains, pure oil from beans, salt from natural sea salt, and sugar from canes. Advanced methods also synthesize several refined foods into one product. When we eat refined food, we digest it within a couple of hours or even faster, using lots of enzymes produced by our body rather than the food's natural enzymes (which act slower).

One good example is starch. The starch in raw food is stored in hard, compact granules, which are difficult to digest quickly. During cooking at high temperatures, water and heat cause the starch granules to expand, burst, and free up individual molecules. This is how gravy is made—by heating flour and water until the starch granules burst and the gravy thickens. Cooking starchy food makes it much easier and faster to digest, but this also creates challenges for the body.

Quickly digested food is broken down into simple sugar, which in turn floods the bloodstream. When blood sugar peaks, the pancreas releases insulin to store energy and to convert unused energy to fat. Insulin also inhibits the burning of already existing fat. When there is a sharp increase of blood sugar, a lot of insulin is released by the body. The insulin does its work and makes the blood sugar drop. But this sudden drop in blood sugar then makes us hungry and we crave more food. Thus, an accelerated digestion of food causes three unhealthy patterns:

- High insulin assists conversion of sugar into fat and inhibits the burning of fat.
- The quick drop of blood sugar, due to a violent insulin response, generates a craving for more food and thus more calorie intake. The cycle continues.
- Fast digestion makes the body adapt to eating food that has no enzymes of its own. The body makes up the difference

and becomes a digestive-enzyme-making machine. This not only reduces the amount of enzymes that are available to other metabolic functions but it also speeds up the depletion of our total enzyme potential.

On the other hand, when we eat foods that are digested more slowly, we reverse these unhealthy patterns. *Slower digestion, or more precisely, a slower release of sugar into the bloodstream, makes us less hungry, burns more fat, and teaches the body to wait for the food's own enzymes to take action.*

Eating food that digests slowly also keeps our blood sugar and insulin response as smooth and even as possible. The standard glucose tolerance test (GTT) measures the body's response to an oral dose of glucose. The patient must fast for 12 hours prior to the test. A baseline fasting blood sugar and insulin is measured. Then a glucose-rich drink (glucola) is administered. After ingesting the "cola," blood sugar and insulin are measured at 30, 60, 90, and 120 minutes. The following diagram on the next page, from "The Role of Dietary Carbohydrate in the Decreased Glucose Tolerance of the Elderly," an article published in the 1987 *Journal of American Geriatrics*, shows the typical glucose-insulin response for healthy young people versus old people.

By eating slow-digesting, live-enzyme food and by following a caloric-restricted diet like the one we will describe in the next chapter, a middle-aged person can achieve a fasting glucose between 60 and 85, and then can return to exactly the same level 120 minutes after taking glucola. In comparison, after 120 minutes of the glucola drink, a young healthy individual on a normal diet can only return their glucose levels to 115, a level far higher than their starting baseline glucose of 90 (measured when fasting), as shown in the following figure.

The scientific method of measuring the absorption rate of food into the bloodstream is known as the glycemic index (GI), which is the ratio of absorption rates between a particular food and pure sugar, both containing equivalent amounts of carbohydrates. Pure sugar is the easiest to absorb and therefore has a rating of 100. The index of any food is less or equal

Typical Glucose Tolerance Response

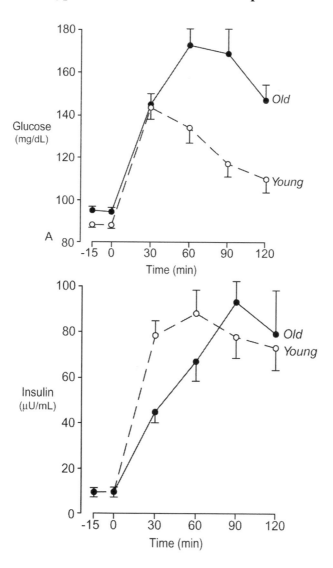

to 100 (%). The higher the index, the quicker the food is absorbed into the bloodstream. *To increase our longevity and our health, we should eat food with a lower glycemic index, the low GI food.* In general, starchy and refined foods have a higher glycemic index because they are easily decomposed into the blood. Below is a list of very low and very high GI foods:

Low and High Glycemic Index Food

Lowest GI Food	GI	Highest GI Food	GI
Apple	38	Bagel	72
Cherries	22	Bran/corn flakes	75-85
Grapefruit	25	Breads	50-95
Pear	38	Crackers	65-87
Plums	39	Potatoes	60-95
Barley	25		
Beans	18-27		
Chana dal	8		
Milk	27		
Soy milk	31		
Yogurt	33		
Peanuts	14		
Rice bran	19		
Pasta/spaghetti	32-40		
Vinegar	0		

What is the function of fat in the body? In nature, animals accumulate fat to keep them from starving. Bears accumulate lots of fat before winter and slowly burn it off during hibernation. Thus, fat is used to store energy during periods of no energy intake.

We need a continuous supply of glucose in the bloodstream to carry out all the body's functions and to supply tissues with energy. During dieting or starvation, when glucose intake is low, the very limited reserves of spare proteins and carbohydrates are broken down to make more glucose. After we use up the glucose in the blood, many tissues switch over to use the products of fat breakdown (known as ketones) as an alternative source of fuel. When glucose is scarce, ketones are produced from fatty tissue and transported through the bloodstream to the liver, where ketone bodies are formed. The ketone bodies are then released into the bloodstream to be taken up and used for energy by the muscles, the heart, the brain, and many other tissues.

Like cars, our bodies can use different types of fuels. Cars use diesel, regular, unleaded, or supreme unleaded gasoline. Regular gasoline burns far less efficiently than supreme grade, leaving more oxidation and waste products inside the car engines. Similarly, burning ketones from fat is a much less efficient process than burning glucose, leaving more oxidants or free radicals in the body. The result: our body ages more.

In a developed nation such as the United States, there is almost always more food than one can consume. Fat in our bodies has, in fact, lost its use. We should be thinner and yet 61% of Americans are overweight. Why? Because the food we eat has a high glycemic index and a high insulin sensitivity. When insulin is high, fat is not burned. A person becomes hungrier and wants to eat more. When there is a constant need to produce a high quantity of insulin, the body either begins to lose the ability to produce more insulin or becomes less effective in binding insulin to cell receptors, resulting in diabetes. Some 10% of Americans are diabetic in their fifties, according to a September 4, 2000 article in *Newsweek* titled "An American Epidemic: Diabetes."

NATURE'S FOURTH LAW OF FOOD

According to the universal law of energy, the higher the frequency at which energy vibrates, the closer it is to the ultimate Tao, the infinite energy source. Applied to humans, the higher one's chi and spirit energy, the more one can "communicate" to the cosmic energy sources to extend their own energy level and life. *Thus, the highest energy source is the subtle energy from the universe. The more we can access and absorb this energy, the more we can preserve our own energy.* Higher beings (people with more pure energy) are able to absorb this higher subtle energy from the universe.

Food produces energy at different levels. We are not just talking about the calories and nutrients for the measurable energy needs of the body but also higher subtle energy forms that modern technology is not capable of measuring. To repeat, cooked food has less of this higher energy than raw, fresh, or live food. These live foods receive energy from the universe (for example, in the form of sunlight, which is yang energy) and from the earth (such as in the form of nutrients, which is yin energy) and synthesize them into energy that humans can absorb.

In turn, live food has less energy than direct cosmic energy, such as sunlight, moonlight, high-energy air, high-energy water, and the infinite energy of the universe. Most of us have not developed the ability to directly absorb such energies fully, but the more we are able to do so, the less we need to depend solely on food for our energy needs.

Both water and air are important carriers of energy. For example, a homeopathic pill is made by dissolving herbs into water and diluting the solution until no herbal molecules remain. The resulting homeopathic remedy contains only water molecules without any chemical trace of herbs. How, then, is the remedy effective?

The water is actually modulated to the herbs' vibrational frequencies. If the herbs are tuned to the frequency of the energy centers of the body (a topic we will take up later), using the modulated water would potentially help heal the body.

Similarly, some chi-gong masters use their hands to emit chi into water and then send the water to remote patients for healing. Very high-energy water, such as spring water directly from high mountains, absorbs a lot of cosmic energy. The more spiritually developed you are (and thereby more attuned to higher frequencies), the more you are able to absorb energy from high-energy water.

Air is another important energy source. High-energy air is air that is charged with negative ions and cosmic energy. The negative ions are now measurable by modern instruments; cosmic energy is yet to be measured.

Modernization has eliminated most high-energy water and air from our environment. Waters are polluted, treated, and recirculated. In large office buildings, shopping malls, and factories, air is usually de-ionized through filters and air conditioning. Fresh air is neutralized through windows with metal frames and screens. Dead air is recirculated over and over again. Smog from traffic and industrial pollution also neutralizes the air. Not only does pollution poison the body, but this dead air carries little higher energy.

We talk about getting "re-charged" when we spend time by the ocean or in the mountains. Ocean or mountain breezes make you feel "charged" because of the high energy of the air, which contains large amounts of negative ions. Polluted air has clusters with positive electricity, which neutralize the negative ions. Negative ions increase our energy levels and help clean the body. In fact, studies show that the human body resembles a semiconductor, which conducts electricity under certain conditions. Air that is high in negative ions literally charges the body.

Another component of high-energy air is oxygen. When the percentage of oxygen in air is high, the body is required to perform less work and our respiratory processes are therefore more efficient. Over the course of a lifetime, this efficiency makes a huge difference.

Thus, the energy in air depends on the level of negative ionization, the percentage of oxygen, the percentage of pollutants, and the percentage of higher energies it carries. The more time we spend in an environment that has pure, high-energy air and water, the more higher energy we can absorb into our bodies.

In later chapters, we will introduce methods of alchemy that can purify and refine your energy so that you can learn to absorb more energy directly from universal sources of energy, such as sunlight and pure air, and reduce the quantity of calories you take in.

In summary, food has three values to humans: (1) calories to burn to produce energy for work, such as thinking and walking; (2) nutrition to nourish the body for such things as building and repairing tissues; and (3) higher level energy, the chi, to sustain life.

All natural foods in their raw living states have these three values. Modern processed foods, however, are high in calories but low in nutrition and energy. When we eat a lot of processed food, we tend to eat more because the value of the food cannot satisfy our body's needs. And we grow larger because the extra calories we take in easily form fat.

Most people have to depend totally on physical food because they do not have the ability to absorb cosmic energy. However, more highly developed beings can partially or completely depend on water, air, and cosmic energy (rays). Not only is this a much more efficient use of energy, thus extending life, but the higher frequency energy can also enhance our life in other ways.

APPLYING THE PROTOCOL

It is clear from this chapter that we need to train our bodies back to nature and follow the laws of nature's food as well as the universal law of energy. The most efficient high-energy foods have the following characteristics: *they are live, raw, high nutrition, low calorie, low glycemic index, and high subtle energy.*

The more you can incorporate these foods into your diet, the longer, healthier, and happier you will be. You will lose unwanted weight, gain considerable energy, and get back your youthful body shape.

The following table shows how you can use and enjoy these types of foods in your daily meals.

Longevity Food	Recipes – No Cooking
raw vegetables raw seaweeds sun-dried vegetables	Eat sun-dried vegetables with homemade salad dressings (see below). You will grow to like the vegetables plain after you develop a taste for the natural flavor.
raw sugar raw honey raw cold pressed oil raw vinegar lime juice raw sea salt raw chili powder other raw seasonings	Use to make sauces and dressings. Try different combinations of sweet, sour, salt, etc. You will be amazed at how many delightful flavors you can create.
raw fruits raw fruit juice sun-dried raw fruits	Use juices that are not pasteurized. Eat fruits at least one hour away from your main meal.

raw deep ocean fish raw deep ocean shellfish low-temp dried/smoked fish raw bean sprout any kind of tofu plain roasted nuts protein supplements	These are your protein sources. Avoid any farm-fed animals, including fish. Use "sushi" grade raw fish. Use the ingredients listed above to create dressings. Roast nuts to unlock enzyme inhibitors. When taking protein supplements, choose the ones with digestive enzymes.
raw baby corn/grains	Eat when the corn is young and milky inside.
raw yogurt raw milk raw butter raw cheese	Use instead of pasteurized diary products. They taste better and are more nutritious.
natural spring water high-energy clean air	Very important. With high-energy air and water, you will need less food and will have a cleaner and more efficient body.
Top quality multi-vitamins & minerals	A good daily supplement to our diets. Even with high-energy food, we cannot be sure if it was grown in soil and water that was rich in vitamins and minerals.

Less Desirable Food	Comments
rice bread pasta spaghetti cooked vegetables cooked beans	Try to eat less of these foods. Use high-quality *pre-meal plant-based digestive enzymes* right before the meal to preserve your own enzymes. If you cannot control craving, take insulin-sensitivity-reducing herbs to reduce appetite.
whole grain bread whole wheat bread deeply cooked food greasy food highly starchy food highly refined food highly processed food packaged food canned food	Skip 1-2 meals after eating a large meal of "less desirable" foods to let the body clean itself. Eat less artificially raised chicken, beef, and fish, which may be grown with hormones, and less food grown in unnaturally short periods of time.

ROAST NUTS AND SEEDS

As a reminder, raw seeds and nuts contain natural substances that allow them to be stored. These enzyme inhibitors lock enzyme actions unless placed in warm and moist conditions. When a food's enzymes are locked, the food can be very upsetting to the stomach, which must work extra hard to digest it, using its own body-produced enzymes. Instead of conserving our enzymes, we use up extra enzymes. The key is to avoid raw nuts and seeds. They must be roasted or sprouted in order to be easily digestible.

VITAMIN AND MINERAL SUPPLEMENTS

Another point to clarify is the use of vitamin and minerals. Today many fruits and vegetables are grown in soils that have been overused for many years. According to the latest U.S. Department of Agriculture food tables, there has been a huge decrease in the nutritional value of food over the last 40 years. Taking spinach as an example, its content of vitamin C has been reduced by 45%, Vitamin A by 17.1%, calcium by 6.5%, potassium by 18.7%, and magnesium by 10.2%.

Because of the depletion of the soil in which our food is grown, it is important to supplement our diets with the appropriate multivitamins and minerals. It is also good to supplement our diets with wild fruits, vegetables, and seaweeds, which contain much higher nutritional values.

MAKING THE TRANSITION

You may wonder if you can follow the kind of diet described above. The idea is to take one step at a time. Try to be creative. If you are not able to eat all of these foods raw, start by using the raw ingredients to make healthy sauces and seasonings. You don't have to use any specific recipes. Make dishes that suit your own taste.

There is a notion that raw food is hard to digest. This is generally not correct. Except for foods that have enzyme inhibitors in their raw state, which we should definitely avoid, we *want* our food to digest more slowly (in accordance with the natural laws of food). This will allow the food's own decomposing enzymes to take effect instead of wasting our precious enzyme reserves and overworking our digestive system.

To begin the transition to better foods, you can also avoid eating refined foods and those with a high glycemic index. At times you may still want to eat "junk" food. Do so to satisfy your body, but always take pre-meal enzymes, use insulin-sensitivity-reducing herbs (to reduce the meal's glycemic index), and skip or lighten the next meals so that your system can clean itself out completely right away.

Make sure that when you eat, your "stomach" is completely empty (you will feel hungry). Gradually, you will find yourself adapting to cleaner, more energetic food over just a few months. You will crave less and less food in the "less desirable" category. Let the transition take place naturally. There is no need to force yourself.

If you're still not convinced about the practical benefits of eating according to nature's original design, read the next chapters for even more compelling reasons to start.

CHAPTER 4

SECOND PROTOCOL: MAXIMIZE METABOLIC EFFICIENCY

"I used to be very proud of my body—lean and muscular," said Eric, an old friend from high school. "But since I turned 35, I've gained 15 pounds and a belly. I lost the beautiful muscle tone, too, and now tire easily. Guess it's time to admit that I'm middle aged and have to forget the body."

"Are you sure you have lost muscle?" I asked. "I think your young physique is still there, perhaps hiding under a layer of fat covering the muscles."

"Well, you're actually right. I tried to lose weight a couple of times on some program and by doing a lot of exercises. I got back in good shape for a short period. But as soon as I relaxed the routine, the pounds started adding on again. How can anyone be expected to live on powders and boring exercise forever? And how come I look and feel so big yet fall into the appropriate range of the recommended normal body weight index?"

While waiting for my reply, Eric popped a whole Reese's peanut butter cup into his mouth.

"That body weight index is based on the average of the whole American population. Being within the range does not mean you are healthy and fit, because you have your own genes. Your best weight is the weight you had when you were young, around 20. There are ways to eat the foods you like and also get your weight back to where you were. You will not feel hungry. You will have lots of energy and get your muscular toned body back without the extreme exercises."

"Really?"

"Let's try it."

Six months later

"Ping, it's amazing! I'm lean and energetic," said Eric enthusiastically. "I play basketball with these very competitive 20-something guys and feel like running all the time."

"Are you compromising your cravings?"

"No. On the contrary, since I'm fit and know how to maintain it, I can sometimes eat things that I had to force myself away from before—butter, cake, chocolate. Your program has helped me get my freedom back."

"There is another huge benefit," I said slowly.

"What is it?" Trying to hurry me up, Eric grabbed my arm.

"Consuming only about one-third of the calories you took in before going on this protocol will extend your life span. Not only will you feel better, but I'd say you'll look 40 at age 60. You probably can live a third longer, too."

"How can that be?" he wondered.

"Just think about your car," I said, employing an analogy I often use. "It can run about 150,000 miles. At 20 miles per gallon, this is about 7,500 gallons of gasoline used for its entire life. The sooner you burn up all the gas, the quicker the car gets old. For people, it is the same thing. The quicker we burn calories, the faster our body parts get rusty. If you burn calories at one-third the rate of others, isn't that going to reduce your rate of aging? "

Ping's Diary

Metabolism represents all of the body's chemical processes, growth, repair, and digestion. It is divided into anabolic (the growth and repair) process and catabolic (decomposition) process, and is indirectly related to heart rate, body temperature, caloric intake, etc. Metabolic rate is defined as calories burned per gram of body mass per day. It is basically a measure of how fast you live—the rate of living.

This protocol will ask you to lower your metabolic rate, and one very effective way of lowering metabolic rate is through caloric restriction. Thus, we will concentrate in this chapter on the benefit and methods of caloric restriction.

You may immediately wonder why we want it lower. Don't all the advertisements talk about accelerating metabolic rate to burn fat and get you back in shape? Aren't many anti-aging clinics offering growth hormone and related therapy to increase your anabolic rate (thus metabolic rate) to stimulate cell growth? Even herbalists talk about how the Chinese herbs accelerate metabolic rate. The topic requires more in-depth study because it is critical to health and longevity.

Metabolic rate is the rate of living: how fast you live through your limited life potential. You can walk 100 miles in less or longer time, depending on the pace. Conceptually, if you live at a faster rate, you end your life sooner, given that you only have a finite capacity to live, according to the law of life.

Think about cars again. A car may run for 150,000 miles before the engine dies. You can maintain your car by changing oil, tuning up the engine, replacing brakes. But it still has a finite number of miles to run. If you burn gas to run faster, the car will break down sooner. Why? The reason is that burning gas or cleaning the engine is never 100% effective. There are always deposits, oxidization, and rust plus mechanical wear and tear.

Similarly, people burn fuel with the aid of the oxygen they breathe. The process is not 100% efficient. The by-product when burning fuel (glucose) with the aid of oxygen gradually kills the living body systems through oxidation as the repair mechanism becomes less and less effective. The reason older people look different from younger ones has to do with damage in the proteins of the body through oxidation over a lifetime.

Proteins are most responsible for the daily functioning of living organisms. Many researchers over the last decade verified that protein modification is a major pathway for aging and degenerative diseases, and one of the major processes that destroys proteins is glycation. Glycation occurs when proteins react with sugars. Then, through a series of reactions, including oxidation, advanced glycation and products (the so-called AGEs) form. AGEs accelerate aging processes and promote degenerative disease. This is the equivalent of browning food in the oven—and equally irreversible.

Science has discovered that the higher the metabolic rate, the lower the maximum life span among mammals. The book *The Biology of Aging*, edited by J.A. Behnke, et al., 1978, reported a research result by Richard G. Culter demonstrating the relationship between maximum life-span potential and specific metabolic rate for some common mammals, as shown in the following diagram.

Relationship between Maximum Life Span and Metabolic Rate for Mammals

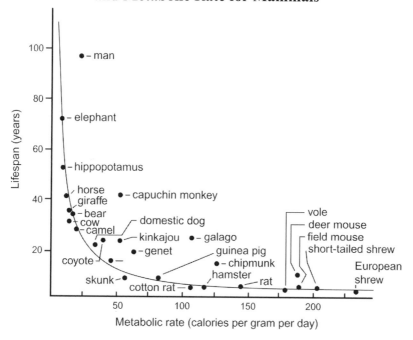

For example, a dog's metabolic rate, or calories burned per gram of body mass per day, is about two times that of man. A dog's maximum life span is about one sixth of man's.

Non-mammals have a similar phenomenon between life span and metabolic rate. A well-known scientific study on worms, published in the *Proceedings of the National Academy of Sciences of the United States of America* in 1999, shows that longevity is increased when the metabolic rate goes down and vice versa. Mutations of the soil worm that increase its longevity could define which specific genes are involved in the aging process. The actions from these gene mutations could reduce animal metabolic rate and, consequently, increase longevity. Environmental conditions that reduce the worm's metabolic rate also extend longevity. It was found that the metabolic rate of long-lived mutations is reduced compared with that of worms found in the wild. However, when a certain gene was "turned off," it restored normal longevity and higher metabolic rate to the long-lived mutants. Thus the increased longevity may result from lowering their metabolic rate rather than an alteration of a genetic pathway that leads to enhanced longevity.

Another non-mammal example, with a life span of over 150 years in polar climates, is the fresh water pearl mussel— margaritifera margaritifera—one of the longest-lived animals on earth. An ongoing study of the species is being conducted by scientists at the Institute of Developmental Biology in Moscow in order to generate genetic and physiological mechanisms contributing to longevity.

The study compares six southern populations in Spain, with maximum-recorded ages of 28-40 years, to three Arctic populations in northwest Russia, with maximum ages of 116-155 years. Within Arctic populations, 20% of mussels live more than 90 years in rivers that are pristine. Possible evolutionary significance of northern longevity is an adaptation to severe cold and unstable environments in high gradient rivers. During winter, mussels have a near famine existence during the Polar Night.

In response, northern populations have much lower metabolic rates, reducing energy expenditure for growth under normal as well as extreme conditions. However, this species is capable of increasing its metabolic rate up to 130 times for tissue regeneration and self-healing.

As we will discuss later in this chapter, caloric restriction is the most effective way of reducing metabolic rate. However, in the modern world, we do the opposite—dramatically increase our caloric intake and thus our metabolic rate.

In sum, *vibrant health and long young life is associated with a much more reduced long-term metabolic rate. The most effective way to reduce metabolic rate is to restrict calories.*

THE OBESITY EPIDEMIC

The last decade of the twentieth century has been dubbed the Fat Decade. With a swiftness that alarmed public health experts, the number of adult Americans considered obese soared during the 1990's to nearly 20%, and the number of those who are overweight has increased to 61% of the population according to the 2000 survey by the U.S. Centers of Disease Control and Prevention. The agency calls the rise in obesity an "epidemic."

Even in the context of constant warnings about the nation's bulging waistline, the findings are stunning. They come in the face of growing knowledge about the risk of being overweight and a steady stream of public health messages about the benefits of exercise and low-fat diets. And they raise disturbing prospects that the nation faces an ever-increasing prevalence of diabetes, cardiovascular disease, and other health problems associated with obesity.

"We don't use the word epidemic lightly," said Jeffrey P. Koplan, director of the CDC. "This is an unexpected rapid increase in the number of cases of obesity and it's really remarkable. Indeed, the speed of the increase was characteristic not of chronic conditions, but of communicable diseases like the flu."

The increase in obesity was found across age and gender groups and geographic regions, suggesting "that there have been sweeping changes in U.S. society that are contributing to weight gain." The highest increases occurred in people between 18 and 29 years old and in those with at least some college education.

Public health officials measure weight using a body-mass index (BMI), defined as the metric weight divided by the square of the metric height. Obesity is defined as a BMI of 30 or over. Generally, people with a BMI of between 25 and 29.9 are considered overweight. A "normal" BMI is 19 to 24.9.

PingLongevity defines the ideal weight to be what you weigh at 18-22 years old. It is *your* ideal rather than someone else's ideal average. Any weight over your ideal is due to more calories taken in than burned up.

Calorie requirement drops as people age because we aren't growing (unless it's a belly) any more and we don't exercise as much. But consumption of calories usually does not fall. We tend to eat as much even when we are not that hungry. We still keep a teenage schedule of three meals and two snacks a day. Thus we consume more calories than we can burn and we put on weight.

Many of us were led to believe that if we don't eat fat, we won't gain weight. However, all foods have their caloric values, such as protein, fat, or carbohydrates. If your calorie intake (not just the amount of fat) is more than you need, the food will be converted to fat or semi-digested gunk. There are vegetarians who are overweight because they eat too many carbohydrates—more than the body can consume.

When you take in more calories than necessary, there are only a few ways to deal with it. The body has to burn the calories through an equal amount of converted work (exercise, labor). It can also convert the calories into fat to store in the body.

There is a third way to deal with the excess calories. When a person consumes more than necessary and continues to gain weight due to stored fat, the body becomes less efficient, even in making fat. Our weight cannot grow infinitely, so the body starts to store "junk," things that are toxic and foreign. The body also becomes a non-productive machine. It uses enzymes and energy to try to digest food. The semi-digested food is also largely expelled from the body. Thus, you waste energy and enzyme potential on harmful work.

The obese often engage in an intensive exercise program. They hire the best trainers. They sweat, lifting weights. They may even burn some fat or consume the extra calories to keep fat constant. But they cannot keep up with the hard regime and so put the fat back on.

They then try something different. They grab one of the fad diets and eat powder mix for a few weeks to lose weight. It works, except it cannot be sustained forever. So they gain the fat back.

Three bad side effects can occur. First, as discussed earlier, fat is a very inefficient fuel source for the body. It generates more by-products of oxidants, which accelerate aging. As you burn fat, you age faster. Second, you go through fat and lean cycles, and your skin has to adapt to larger or smaller sizes. Your skin loses elasticity after the mid-30's, and you appear older than you are. Third and most importantly, the body simply does not need, nor can it use up, the intake of extra calories.

The fact is, we burn many less calories than when we were growing, yet we still keep the habit of eating three meals and two desserts a day and consume the same amount we did as a youngster.

Let's again talk about the car analogy. Imagine that your car used to run 40 miles a day to commute to work and needed a full tank of gas once a week. Now you have changed jobs, drive only 10 miles a day, and don't need as much gas. Yet you run your car at idle for five hours every day so you can still use up a full tank of gas once a week. Isn't it silly? But this is exactly what you do to yourself when taking in more calories than you need.

In conclusion, storing fat—nature's protection against severe conditions such as freezing temperatures or lack of food—is unnecessarily used in modern society as a daily endeavor. The body will adapt. If you want it to be simply a digestion machine, it will. When the body is overfed, it runs dirtier inside and becomes less efficient.

CALORIC RESTRICTION

Caloric restriction without malnutrition is the only scientifically recognized method to expand life. It extends the maximum life span, delays and reduces degenerative diseases, and dramatically slows aging.

Let's look at a few scientific experiments.

There are many animal studies showing the effect of calorie restriction on maximum life span. The first report was by Professor Clyde McCay of Cornell University in 1935, showing that animals on a caloric restriction far outlived animals allowed to eat as much as they wanted.

Studies on rats conducted by Dr. Roy Walford at the UCLA School of Medicine in 1986 also demonstrated the dramatic improvement of life span. Rats have a maximum life span of around 35 months, equivalent to a human's 120 years. Every 10 months of a rat's lifetime is about 34 years of a human. Experiments have shown that a 10% restriction of calories can delay a rat's aging and maximum life span by 10 months, equivalent to about 34 years in a human. A 50% restriction delays aging by 18 months in rats, equivalent to about 60 years in a human.

This is an increase of maximum life span by 50%. Since disease is usually associated with aging, a delay of aging by 50% is an extension of young life.

Monkeys resemble humans more than rats do but are difficult to study because of their longer life span. A long-term groundbreaking primate study is being conducted by a team of scientists led by Dr. R. Weindruch at the University of Wisconsin-Madison. A preliminary report was published by Jennifer Christensen and Richard Weindruch, "Calorie Restriction in Monkeys" in *Life Extension,* July 1998.

Monkey experiments show that a 26% reduction in calorie intake can result in 0.5°F reduction in body temperature, 28% reduction in glucose, 77% reduction in insulin, 30% reduction in weight, 66% reduction in body fat, and 400% increase in insulin sensitivity. High insulin sensitivity is a sign of high metabolic efficiency—similar to a highly efficient car engine.

The data is summarized in the following table:

Monkey Experiment on Caloric Restriction

Normal Diet	Reduced Diet
Food intake daily: 662 calories	Food intake daily: 488 calories
Body weight: 31.5 pounds	Body weight: 20.5 pounds
Body fat: 26%	Body fat: 8.6%
Abdominal measure: 24.4 inches	Abdominal measure: 16.5 inches
Body mass: 47.6 (kg/m^2)	Body mass: 34.2 (kg/m^2)
Basal glucose: 74	Basal glucose: 53
Basal insulin: 44	Basal insulin: 10
Insulin sensitivity: 1.8 (x10^{-4})	Insulin Sensitivity: 9.1 (x10^{-4})
Leptin: 5.8 (ng/milliliter)	Leptin: 1.0 (ng/milliliter)

Human experiments are even more difficult. In 1988, the first man-made full biosphere project was conducted in Tucson, Arizona, with eight people enclosed in a sealed environment. They lived with their own air, plants, environment, animals, and natural resources without outside help. The eight scientists participated in a caloric restriction program for the next six months, eating an 1800-calorie-per-day whole food diet (compared with an average 2500 calorie American diet). The results were published in the *Annuals of Academy of Sciences*, a remarkable improvement in health:

- 15% reduction of weight
- 24% lower blood sugar

- 38% lower cholesterol
- 30% reduction of blood pressure
- 27% reduction of white blood cell count

Biosphere 2 Experiment
(on eight biospherans before and after 6 months)

	Body Weight		Blood Sugar		Cholesterol		Blood Pressure	
	Before	After	Before	After	Before	After	Before	After
1	208	158	105	82	215	129	100/70	80/50
2	148	135	81	77	145	100	100/70	90/60
3	148	126	89	60	196	107	110/72	70/40
4	150	127	99	72	190	125	135/90	110/70
5	165	142	101	69	209	122	110/80	100/60
6	130	115	77	68	146	83	100/60	80/40
7	123	111	101	68	231	168	110/80	90/60
8	116	100	80	73	199	119	110/70	85/50
Ave	148	126	92	70	191	119	109/77	76/57
chg		15%		24%		38%		30/27%

Many people who measure in the "normal" range are really not healthy. A blood sugar level near 100 is not as good as 70 to 80. The blood is much thicker with sugar, and it deposits into the tissue and blood vessels much faster. So don't stop when a doctor says you're "normal." You must achieve *vibrant health*.

Cancer is the result of an accumulation of toxins, oxidation of body systems, and degeneration of energy potential. Caloric restriction is proven to delay aging, extend maximum life span, and thus greatly reduce cancer. A few experiments performed on rats at the UCLA School of Medicine have shown the incidence of various spontaneous cancers in mice on a calorie-restricted diet compared with normally fed mice.

Cancer	% in normal fed	% in restricted fed
Breast	40	2
Lung	60	30
Leukemia	65	10
Liver	64	11

The calorie-restricted group also had cancer 8-12 months later than the normal fed group. This is equivalent to 15-30 years of a human's life. Extending youthful life free of cancer by 15-30 years is a wonderful thing for anyone.

The life span of many mammalian species is related to the average weight of the adult brain and the average weight of the adult body, a relationship called the index of cephalization. The heavier the brain, as compared to the body weight, the more long-lived a species will be. This relationship, first reported in 1910, was independently rediscovered in 1955 and refined for mammals by the late gerontologist George Sacher.

Experiments have compared farm-raised rats, which were normally fed, to wild rats, which went through fast and feast in the wilderness. It took the farm rats 70 days to reach a body weight of 270g, at which point their brains each weighed 1.7g. However, it took the wild rats 318 days to reach 270g with brain weights of 2.3g. This is a four-times slower aging rate and 35% larger brain for the same body size, showing the important benefit of caloric restriction.

HORMONES

We hear a lot nowadays in the press and advertisements about growth hormone (HGH), testosterone, androgen, DHEA, replacement, and stimulants. Why is the growth hormone level at age 35 less than at age 15? Is that bad?

Not necessarily. At age 15, you still have to grow taller and larger, so you need more HGH. At age 35, you are past maturity size, so the HGH level should be lower. In fact, someone with a pituitary tumor, causing a higher than normal secretion of HGH, will experience bone thickening and develop oversized hands and feet, seen in hypersomatotropism.

Let's ask a different question. Why should the growth hormone level at age 50 be less than at 25? Is that bad? Definitely. This is a sign of old age. Ideally, your growth hormone level should stay at the same level it was when you reached maturity. Some doctors want to add HGH into the bloodstream after you are 50 to keep its levels from dropping. However, the problem is that the total balance of the hormonal system in the body is complicated. It is not possible to balance it by outside body controls. Therefore, externally administrated hormones may cause many side effects and may even increase the risk of cancer.

To illustrate the difficulty of balancing hormones, let's look at diabetes patients who must take insulin daily. Insulin suppresses the blood sugar level from going too high in response to food intake. But our blood sugar level depends on many factors. If you sleep for an hour less, eat an extra apple, climb several stairways, and endure emotional pressure, these will all change blood sugar levels.

So how much insulin do you need for blood sugar not to be too high (in which case the sugary blood clogs all the little veins, such as in the eyes) or too low (in which case you simply pass out)? There is no fixed answer to that question. That is why a diabetic needs to keep a consistent lifestyle.

Sex hormones such as testosterones have similar properties as other hormones. They peak at puberty, gradually come down to a maturity level, and significantly decrease after late middle age, around age 50. Therefore you lose sexual ability and vitality, a sign of lost energy potential. Again, it is difficult to balance externally administrated hormones, which may produce significant long-term side effects.

Caloric restriction has several effects on hormones such as HGH and testosterone. It keeps the hormones at a constant level much longer. It also keeps the body running much more efficiently. Because of a reduced metabolic rate, it takes less hormone secretion to create the same effect. Thus, caloric restriction has the effect of automatically resolving this dilemma of late middle and old age.

. Taking testosterone as an example, scientists have published several reports showing the effect of caloric restriction on rats. Male rats were divided into two control groups, one with 50% caloric restriction and the other with normal food intake. Results are shown in the following graph.

The Effect of Caloric Restriction on Hormones[*]

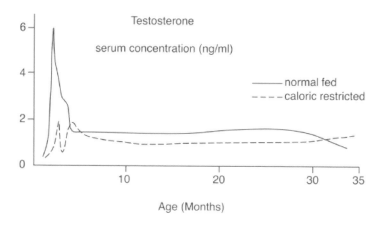

Age (Months)

---

[*] Adapted from: Merry, B.J., & Holehan, A.M., "Serum profiles of LH, FSH, testosterone and 5-alpha-DHT from 21 to 1000 days of age in ad libitum fed and dietary restricted rats." *Experimental Gerontology*, 16: 431, 1981.

Rats in the calorie-restricted group showed a 20-day delay (or 2 1/2 years in a human) in pubertal peak of serum testosterone, a 30% lower testosterone level at the peak, and constant testosterone levels throughout life as opposed to the normally fed group's hormone level declining with age.

The meaning of the chart is significant. Not only is maturity delayed (and thus according to the law of living, aging is delayed), but active sexual life and other benefits of testosterone are extended.

ATHLETIC PERFORMANCE AND IMMUNE FUNCTION

Among other benefits of caloric restriction are athletic performance and immune function. Normally fed and calorie- restricted mice were given a logrolling test. Mice in the calorie-restricted group at age 32 months (about 100 years for a human) could perform logrolling as if they were 12 months old (equivalent to a human's 35). However, from the normal fed group, 32-month-old mice fell off the roller almost every time.

Many scientific experiments have proved that caloric restriction increases immune system capability. Not to burden you with too much scientific data, we present a case study from John, age 38. At age 33 he started putting on weight, mostly in the belly, because he dramatically reduced the calories he burned when active in competitive sports. He had also stopped growing. Coinciding with the period of weight gain, John had a stressful job and started developing a chronic dry cough. The cough was constant throughout the day and subsided during the night when he slept. It was extremely bothersome and embarrassing because he could not speak continuously.

John went through referral after referral to lung, throat, and allergy specialists and underwent many tests, including blood tests, X rays, and ultrasound. Nothing revealed the source of the problem. He even went to the emergency room once, near death, because of an allergic reaction to a doctor-prescribed codeine medication for his "allergy."

Finally, the doctors declared him okay. But, like many people who suffer pain, it does not matter what doctors say; it matters that patients feel pain. John's cough lasted more than one year. John started using the *PingLongevity* protocols. He lost weight and returned to his teenage figure. Surprisingly, corresponding to this timing, his cough went away. He felt energized and came back to his former healthy self.

USING AND PRESERVING ENERGY

Some scientists believe that caloric restriction likely operates through basic and universal mechanisms having to do with energy utilization. All organisms need energy to survive. Depending on their niche, they take energy from many different environmental sources, such as air, water, soil, plants, and animals they eat. To be successful in their evolution, each organism must also develop finely tuned responses for gauging the availability of energy to determine how much they should consume, when it should be consumed, and what should be stored for later use. Based on patterns of energy consumption, responses are made that determine growth and reproduction as well as further food-seeking behavior.

For many organisms, like C. elgans, a kind of worm, expectation of low energy availability, triggered by overpopulation, produces a dormant stage of development called the dauer larva. In this form, the organism is small and reproductively immature but can withstand environmental stressors and can live many weeks longer than it typically does. When the energy environment is more favorable, the organism reverts to its normal form and continues to develop and mature, and then finally shows signs of aging and dies. There are many invertebrates with similar strategies for dormancy. In mammals, a possible parallel strategy is hibernation.

While caloric restriction does not produce a dauer larva or a formal state of hibernation in mammals, many gerontologists are intrigued by the parallels and the evolutionary significance of this strategy. We can consider that the mammalian response to caloric restriction follows a similar strategy (although it does not go as far as some species) because of the remarkable parallels between the physiological effects of caloric restriction and those of hibernation, among them reduced blood glucose, insulin, and white blood cell counts.

Recent genetic studies have shed light on the possibility that caloric restriction might operate through a pathway similar to that which controls the formation of the dauer larva. Several genes have been identified that promote longevity. When the expression of one of these genes is reduced or mutated, the worm can enter the dauer stage, exhibiting a nearly doubled life span compared to worms with the normal gene.

It may be true that the vital essence (the prenatal chi we have at birth, stored mostly in the adrenal gland) is proportional to the rate that calories are burned by the body.

Again, eat less, live longer.

ADULT-ONSET DIABETES

It would be interesting to examine the process of adult-onset diabetes because it is an amplified case of the overconsumption of calories. It is a degenerative disease that is rapidly growing in industrialized countries.

Food is converted into blood sugar. The purpose of insulin is to keep the sugar in the blood at normal levels. Soon after we eat food, our blood sugar level goes up. In response, the pancreas releases insulin. As insulin binds on the cells' receptors, it allows sugar to pass from the bloodstream into the body's cells to be used as fuel. Extra blood sugar is converted into fat. In the case of adult-onset diabetes, although the pancreas may produce insulin, the body is insensitive to the insulin action, thus keeping a high blood sugar level.

When blood sugar remains constantly high, the blood becomes thicker, stickier, and less fluid. Just think about pure water as compared with sugary water. It is harder for thicker blood to travel through small blood vessels, such as those in the eyes and the extremities. When these areas cannot be nourished, and toxins cannot be carried away by the blood, functional failures result. For example, that is why diabetics may have eye problems. In addition, thicker blood becomes sticky, depositing itself on the walls of blood vessels. It builds up, narrows the pathways, and pollutes the blood circulation system.

A high blood sugar level also causes protein-glucose complexes—medically called AGE (advanced glycosolation endproducts)—a form of cellular garbage that accumulates with age and interferes with the workings of the cells. Excess glucose in the blood cross-links with and damages proteins. As more and more proteins are damaged, the body gets old.

Adult-onset diabetes often goes hand in hand with being overweight. Besides genetic reasons (which can play an important role but are not the whole picture), it starts with overeating. When we constantly eat too much over a long period of time, the body has to produce a lot of insulin and bind it to the cells. A constantly high insulin level not only depletes the body's reserve to produce insulin hormones but also makes the cells' receptor less sensitive and efficient. Thus, people become overweight and diabetic.

If diabetes that is caused by excessive caloric intake is an example of accelerated aging, caloric restriction is a great way to decelerate aging. As you can see, the real issue has to do with our choice of lifestyle. One is the accelerated rate of living in which we age much faster and get into the age-related degenerative diseases earlier. The other is a decelerated rate of living. It is our choice indeed.

APPLYING THE PROTOCOL

There are several questions we need to address. First, exactly how many calories do we need? Second, don't we crave more calories because we naturally need them? Do we need to suffer to have good health?

How many calories do we need? There are only two tests. Do you keep a constant weight and do you feel energetic? The intake of calories must be no more than the calories burned. If you take in more calories than you burn, the calories have no place to go but to add to your weight. Therefore, the best measure of caloric intake is your weight.

You don't have to count calories. It should be a closed loop feedback system. You should watch your weight and adjust your calorie intake to keep the weight at the ideal. If you keep the weight at the ideal and make sure of sufficient nutrition, you should always feel energetic. If you lack energy, question your nutrition intake, since we must make sure to restrict caloric intake *without malnutrition*.

What is your ideal body weight? Calorie-counter books will tell you that your ideal weight is your body mass index (BMI), defined as your weight in kilograms divided by the square of your height in meters. They say that if the number is less than 18.5, you are underweight. If it is higher than 25, you are overweight. This is based on statistics of the average population. Nowadays we have many recommended numbers, such as the daily dietary allowance, the normal blood pressure, normal blood sugar levels, and ideal weight. However, these are all based on the range of statistical average. Everyone is genetically different.

A very thin person may be perfectly healthy but way below the average weight. An average weight would be bad for a naturally thin person because it asks for unnatural weight gain. The other bad thing about average ideals is that usually the optimal is at the very low end or high end of the "normal" range. Take blood sugar, for example. The medically recommended blood sugar level is 70-100. If you are 95, you are considered in great shape. However, for what we call *vibrant health*, the super-healthy human, we'd like to see 70-85.

According to the law of life, 18-22 is the peak energy age, when the body is supposed to be in the best physical shape—either heavy or light, depending on genetic makeup. After this age, energy is moving into the down cycle. The key to vibrant health is to delay and slow the down cycle. It is not difficult to conclude that the ideal weight for each individual is the weight of the individual at age 18-22.

In addition to calories, the intake of nutrients, fatty acids, and proteins must be equal to the need of the body. When the intake is too little, it will impair the construction and repair of body parts due to the lack of essential raw materials. When it is right, we always feel an increased energy for restricted caloric intake. Again, when people tire because of reduced caloric intake, it means more nutrition is needed. Therefore, we must consider increasing nutritional contents without increasing calories.

Now let us answer the second question: Don't we crave more calories because we naturally need them? Can we take less calories without being miserable? This seems to be difficult. Here is a quote from an article written by Dr. Stephen Coles of the Los

Angeles Gerontology Research Group in 1996: "Although the causal relation between caloric restriction and maximum life-span extension was discovered as long ago as 1932, even today, it is still the only known intervention, possibly along with pineal cross transplantation, shown to produce such an effect. Yet no one appears willing to use this method to prolong life. Why not? Because people are more interested in the quality of life than in its quantity, and the inconvenience factor of always being hungry makes it prohibitive."

There are several ways of achieving higher quality of life with caloric restriction. *First, eat high-quality nutritious food to maximize the nutrition value per calorie intake.* This way, your intake is more efficient so the body needs less total calories. What is high-quality nutritious food? As we discussed in Chapter 3, it is raw, live, and clean (e.g., food grown with high energy air, water, food, and soil) and is a low glycemic index food.

The second way to restrict calories is to know how to eat a lot of food without consuming a lot of calories. One experiment you can do is to take a bowl of salad or greens, cook it, and see how much is left. Eating a large quantity of raw vegetables equates to a small amount of cooked ones in volume. Now try to eat nuts. A cup of roasted peanuts is approximately 120 calories compared to 250 calories for a medium-sized cone of ice cream or 300 in a single hamburger or 280 in a single chocolate bar. But peanuts will keep you from hunger a lot longer because they have a low glycemic index of 14 and are also very high in protein. Another example is raw milk. A cup of raw milk is many times more efficient than a cup of cooked or pasteurized milk. Thus you need less calories for the same body needs. By eating more foods like this, you can reduce the number of calories you eat each day.

A third way to reduce calories is to use alternative fuel, such as air, cosmic rays, and water, in line with nature's fourth law of food. This requires purifying your spirit and opening up your channels so you can communicate directly with the cosmic energy source.

Fourth, don't burn calories just to be burning them. This is equivalent to burning gas by allowing your car's engine to idle. Extreme exercise wears and tears bones and muscles, accelerates metabolic rate (and the rate of living), and produces no useful work. Light exercise is good without going too far. To reduce weight, the only way is to control caloric input.

If you weigh much more than your ideal weight (your weight at age 18-22), reduce calories (and weight) gradually. Burning fat too fast oxidizes the body too quickly. Be persistent and take many small steps over a 6-12 month period to get down to the ideal weight.

Here is James' story—a real-life example:

"I had been slim, muscular, youthful, healthy, and energetic until I turned 40. Then I gained 25 pounds in two years. I ate as much as I did when I was in my 20's and often felt tired after a day at work. I developed allergies, coughing, sneezing, running nose. I ate mostly Chinese stir-fried food, pork, vegetables, packaged frozen vegetables, tofu, skim milk—thinking I was on a much healthier diet than the usual fast food. But my weight continued to increase and I started to notice my belly. I sometimes stared at old pictures of myself, envying the boyish body, and found myself thinking about my overweight father, uncle, and grandfather having heart diseases, diabetes, and high blood pressure.

"I didn't move like I did as a kid. I needed to reduce calorie intake but got hungry because my body was used to routines. A little further research made me realize that some foods made me hungry the more I ate them, and others made me full for a long time.

"Here is the secret. The same quantity of raw food has about twice the volume as when it is cooked. Also, food like nuts, with a high protein value but very low insulin sensitivity, stuff me full for a long time. Lastly, raw food has more nutritional value for the same quantity. I don't need to take as much raw food as cooked food.

"I started changing my routines while still enjoying food and life. In the morning, I drink two glasses of raw milk bought at a whole food store, plus multivitamin and mineral supplements. The multivitamins and minerals are just for insurance purposes because vegetables and fruits may grow in nutritionally depleted soils, and fast-fed chickens and cows may not be as nutritious as before. Occasionally, I add a little protein powder—the one with digestive enzymes. I drink plenty of green tea (more than 10 cups) throughout the day. I eat a half-cup of roasted peanuts at lunchtime, which stuffs me for the rest of the day.

"Six out of seven nights a week, I eat healthy raw deep ocean fish (tuna), shellfish (oysters), fresh seaweeds (from an Oriental grocery store), raw fresh vegetables (seasoned with uncooked apple cider vinegar, unprocessed honey, and raw sea salt), and tofu. I eat very little starchy food (bread, rice). The more I eat this diet, the less I need flavor. Occasionally, I want junk food— mostly Chinese or Italian at social gatherings. When I do eat junk food, I skip meals the next day to let my body cleanse itself. I can enjoy food and life, and vibrant health too.

"My new scheme turns out to require less than one-fourth of the calories I had in my 20's. Within a few months, I got back to my boyish figure with muscles and no belly. My allergy is gone. I am as energetic as 20 years ago. I play competitive sports with people in their twenties. My life is vibrant again in my 40's."

CHAPTER 5

THIRD PROTOCOL: REDUCE WEARING AND TEARING

Outside everything was completely covered by snow. In the woods, most animals were in their winter hybernation. It was so cold, your breath immediately turned into an icy mist. Inside the university gym, everyone was sweating: laboring on the bicycle machines, watching TV while taking a breather, lifting weights.

After my swimming exercise, I ran into Mary, a research associate.

"Hi, Mary. I didn't know you came here. How are you?"

"Hi, Ping. I come three times a week, as much as I can force myself, trying to follow my doctor's orders," she said, breathing heavily, sweat dripping down her red face, looking like she had just stepped out of a hot oven.

"What orders?" I asked.

"As you can see, I'm overweight. My doctor said I am at high risk of a heart attack and must get my cholesterol, blood pressure, and the fat down. I'm killing myself after a whole day of hard work. My back aches and recently my knee began hurting too. So much pain, and still my weight moves up, never down. My doctor told me exercise is the only way to do it."

Looking around, I saw so many Marys knocking themselves out to lose weight.

"Ping, do you come here often? You stay so slim, you must be here seven days a week."

"No," I said, "I only come a few times a month, mostly to swim."

She looked puzzled and surprised as we said good-bye to each other.

Later, I recalled a doctor saying to me when I was an intern in medical school, "I see so many arthritis patients every day. A lot of their problems are due to forced over-use of their joints, making them wear and tear down sooner. The worst cases come from those who were heavy exercisers or athletes when they were young."

When I started my own medical practice, I began to understand that most people receive double hits—from gaining weight and the wearing of their joints and muscles. There are better ways to control weight than exercises.

Ten years later, I am still in touch with Mary. Now she can't exercise because of severe arthritis and has gained even more weight. Mary seems to have just given up.

Ping's Diary

This chapter will explain how to preserve the body's mechanical systems. By body mechanical system, we mean the physical aspects: bones, muscles, tendons, ligaments, and skin.

When is the first time you feel something wrong with your mechanics? At the first sign of pain. This is the body's way of telling us about problems in our system. How many times have you heard people over age 35 complain about back aches, knee problems, neck pain, hip fractures, muscle strains, nerve pains? The body's mechanics seem to fall apart soon after early middle age. Pain has become one of the modern epidemics. However, it is seldom considered a disease in the medical world if the blood work and X rays come out okay. Usually there is nothing else a doctor can do about it, except prescribe pain killers, which only temporarily suppress the problem.

What is pain? Why isn't it treated as a disease when it is everywhere in our life? Why is it so easy to be in pain but so difficult to cure pain? Besides internal organ malfunctions there are mainly four root causes for the accelerated deterioriation of our body mechanics.

First, bones and muscles are worn out and torn apart by strenuous excercises and the work of a lifetime. Once injured, it is very easy to injure the same area again and again because it is weakened. Injuries hardly ever completely heal or get back to a perfect condition. Over time, we weaken so many of its parts that the entire mechanical system just gets "tired."

Second, when blood and chi are blocked, the right energy and nutrients cannot be sent to some areas of the body, nor the toxins taken away. For example, blood can be too thick because it contains too much sugar or fat. A meridian can be blocked due to long-term emotional issues such as stress. Thick blood (from such things as high sugar and cholesterol) becomes less fluid and more sticky. Compare clear spring water with honey. Try to make them flow through a thin pipe and you will get the idea. There are many small branches of blood vessels, such as in the eyes, kidney, and the extremities, that the blood needs to travel far to reach. When the body parts cannot be nourished sufficiently and waste products cannot be taken away, we experience pain.

Third, kidney, lung, and spleen function has deterioiated. In traditional Chinese medicine, kidney meridian controls the health of the bones, lung meridian governs skin and hair, and spleen meridian dominates muscles. This is consistent with modern science. For example, kidney filters blood, gets rid of waste and toxins, and reabsorbs nutrients and minerals, including calcium and magnesium. Kidneys convert vitamin D into its most biologically active form, 1,25-dihydroxy cholecalciferol, which in turn helps bones use calcium and magnesium. In Chapter 6, we will cover extensively the topic of energy meridian balancing. In traditional Chinese medicine, the kidney system includes sexual organs and functions. Thus, sexual hormones, such as testosterone in men and estrogen in women, have a dramatic influence on keeping the bones, muscles, and skin young. In Chapter 8, we will discuss ways to preserve sexual energy.

A fourth cause for deterioration of body mechanics is the aging of our skin, especially due to exposure to harmful sunrays. The easy way out is to replace the malfunctioned body parts such as hipbones, to stretch the skin to make it look better, and to suck out fat to make us thin. According to statistics tracked by the American Society of Plastic Surgeons, there has been a dramatic increase of plastic surgery procedures in the seven years from 1992 to 1999. Liposuction increased by 389%, breast augmentation by 413%, and eyelid surgery by 139%.

What we want is to stay young naturally. While the new procedures give us options to replace our body parts, nothing is better than natural youthfulness. And there is no sure way to know the side effects of many of the procedures.

We will talk about how to reduce the wearing and tearing of the body parts through a lifestyle change. Then, we will look into the internal organs and energy meridians that balance and nourish the body's mechanics. Finally, we will present easy-to-follow *PingLongevity* protocols.

THE ROLE OF EXERCISE

How much should we exercise? Let us examine two seemingly contradictory claims.

First, it is well known that exercise is good for health. It increases blood circulation, raises the levels of HDL (good cholesterol), lowers blood pressure, improves the immune system, and helps protect the body against many diseases. It reduces the chance of cardiovascular diseases. According to a famous study of 17,000 male alumni of Harvard University between the ages of 35 and 74, those who actively exercised lowered their overall death rates by 25-33% and decreased their risk of coronary artery disease by an astounding 41% when compared with their more inactive fellow alumni. This is easy for us to accept. In fact, it has become fashionable to go to the gym, to hire a personal trainer, and to use exercise to burn fat.

Second, there is an opposing view, not so well publicized. Just take a look at the evaluation process of life insurance companies. Insurance companies make serious money by betting on people's life expectancy. They hire high-powered statisticians to estimate premiums based on the risk of each individual—how he/she will fare according to age, race, health, occupation, family history, and health habits. Professional athletes fall into the high-risk category and command higher premiums for life insurance. According to the American Academy of Orthopedic Surgeons, there were more than three million sports injuries in 1999. A new study at the Duke University Medical Center scanned the knees of 11 basketball players at Duke at the beginning and end of the 1999-2000 season. The magnetic resonance imaging (MRI) snapshots of the knees showed that nearly all of the players had signs of stress, nine out of 22 knees had abnormalities and possible thinning of the cartilage coating the knee bones, and three had jumper's knee—which occurs when the tendon connecting the patella to the tibia, or shinbone, gets inflamed. In some cases, it can degenerate and become disabling.

You can see, on one hand, that exercise is essential to health but, on the other, that it is a serious health risk.

We need to re-address a few key questions: What are the exercises for? Should we exercise as much as possible? Do we really enjoy doing the exercises?

There are several reasons why we exercise:
1. Fun
2. A career (such as athletes)
3. Staying active and healthy
4. Burning fat and looking good

Fun and career are choices. We make choices all the time. We may break bones or develop arthritis due to life-long wear and tear, but it is our choice, and we may think fun and career are worth the risk.

Let's concentrate on the last two reasons: staying active and healthy, and burning fat/looking good.

If we want to stay active and healthy, all we need to do is warm up our blood and pump our heart to improve circulation. This is why there are statistics showing that exercise helps reduce heart disease. But exactly how much is enough to get the blood going? It really depends on your blood. If you have sticky blood (containing too much sugar, fat, toxin), it requires a lot of exercise to get the heart pumping to push the blood through the tiny veins. If your blood is vibrant, fluid, low in fat and sugar, and high in energy, you can achieve good circulation everywhere in the body with meditation alone—no muscle movement! What is wrong with hard exercise? It wears and tears muscles, bones, tendons, and ligaments. It consumes body fluid, such as that in the joints. You know from experience that the more you use your car, the sooner it needs replacement parts.

Exercise for heart and vascular health is inferior to keeping the blood fluid and vibrant through calorie restriction and raw food therapy.

What about burning fat? Burning fat itself is not a fun activity. How many times do we hear co-workers, friends, and relatives complain about how difficult exercise is? If exercises are fun, why do we watch TV while doing them? Most of us want to stay fit. The question, then, is why do we get unfit in the first place?

The old saying is true: work hard, die young. We often get trapped in a dilemma. We know hard labor reduces life span. Yet we put our body (digestive systems and metabolic processes) through hard work whenever we put on weight; then we work even harder to take the fat off through strenuous exercise, weight lifting, treadmills, and marathons. In fact, the more we sweat, the faster we pump our heart, and the harder we work our muscles, the better we think we're doing. This whole cycle is promoted by fashionable fitness programs that push new equipment, electrical stimulation of muscles, supplements to enhance muscle growth, and personal trainers. It has been a passion as well as a fashion. Still, we witness more obesity, and more and more pain! It's time to sit back and think through what we are doing to ourselves.

Let's look to nature for answers. In nature, animals labor to make a living (food and shelter), survive predators, and have playful fun. Otherwise, they usually lie down, rest, and sleep. Just observe your own pets.

For us, fortunately there is much less need to do hard labor. We have machines. We don't need to run away from predators because we are usually well protected. We have fun playing basketball, golf, and tennis. However, we also perform boring tasks for no useful work or fun: lifting weights and walking treadmills. What is the purpose? We are driven to this because we eat too much and need to burn fat. The fat collects under our skin and wraps our organs so we cannot see the beautiful muscle curves of the natural body. Why create the situation in the first place by eating too much— then harm ourselves again by wearing out our mechanical systems through over-exercising?

Exercise is an inefficient way of burning fat and has multiple side effects.

THE HEALTH OF MUSCLE

Like brain cells, muscle cells do not regenerate. Once a muscle cell dies, it cannot be replaced. This is different from skin cells. Once a muscle has been subjected to the stress of misuse or overuse, it cannot repair itself. But like brain cells, muscle cells occasionally are capable of changing function to take over the work of nearby damaged cells. In this way, a person is able to continue walking, running, dancing, and moving, even though some muscle cells might have been damaged over time. The first thing about muscles we have to recognize is that, once damaged, the damage is permanent, although the body can find some other ways for the nearby cells to help. Therefore, we have to be extremely careful not to damage our muscles.

Sports and hard labor definitely increase the chance of muscle damage. For perfect longevity, we prefer light exercises, such as swimming and walking. Light exercise to keep the use of every part of the body is very important to maintain good health. Too much exercise will have negative effects on health. It is against yin-yang principles. The best exercise is tai chi—the ancient Chinese art of movement, which combines mind and body. Yoga is another good exercise.

How about building muscles? We all want to look good, have the right amount of muscles, and the right body lines. Body building is most effective when we are very young. Studies have shown a twofold increase in oxygen metabolism to the muscles during exercise after a brief training session. But while anyone, at any age, can develop stronger and more efficient muscles as a result of exercise training, such conditioning is best begun early in life. The younger you are, the more "trainable" your muscles. Many forces are at work to determine the body shape.

Once muscles are built, they will not be lost until old age. Losing muscle in middle age is a misconception. It is mainly due to the added fat which covers all the body lines and muscles. The reason we lose muscle at old age is not because of a lack of exercises but the degenerated capability of digestion and absorption of nutrients and energy, leading to the body's cannibalizing its own protein reserve.

On the other hand, trying to grow muscle is hard after middle age. It also creates more damage. We don't recommend it. Under a microscope, an aged muscle reveals a loss of cells, atrophy of cells, accumulation of fat and collagen, and loss of contractility. Aging muscles are less flexible than young muscles and are more susceptible to strains, pulls, and cramping. Therefore, *muscle is not replaceable, so never damage it. Muscles are most efficiently trainable between 15-22. Train them young. Engage in only light exercises after 30.*

Traditional Chinese medicine believes the spleen meridian controls muscles. The spleen meridian is the energy system that controls the digestion of nutrients. When the spleen functions normally, the body is adequately nourished; muscles are well developed and limbs are strong. If the spleen's function is impeded, poor appetite results. A prolonged impairment of the spleen can lead to malnutrition, diarrhea, or edema due to retention of water. Hence, the flesh suffers. Thus, *muscles must be nourished by healthy spleen meridian systems. Keep spleen systems balanced and at high energy.* Use the spleen balancing formula discussed in Chapter 6.

THE HEALTH OF SKIN

Maintaining healthy skin is an important part of longevity, not just for a youthful look but because the skin is a very important organ of the body, responsible for many respiratory functions. Skin protects us from environmental changes, cold, hot, harshness, wind, and diseases. Occasionally you meet someone who looks to be 20 but is actually 40. You wonder why. Is it less sun exposure? Not necessarily, because we often find that a person with no suntan has loose facial skin. Is it due to genes? Genes do play a role. But this is always a reassuring excuse for us not to do better. Why, then, is there a big difference between your facial skin and, say, skin on the buttocks?

What indeed drives the health of the skin, especially on the face? Skin is damaged mainly through four common root causes: oxidation, sun UV exposure, weight loss and gain due to feast and fast cycles, and deficient lung energy meridian systems.

Although not well known, much scientific research has gone into the study of cells—what causes a cell to live longer, grow faster when damaged, and divide more times.

As most of us know, whether from the skin or any other organ, all normal cells have a finite life span except for a few exceptions, such as cancer cells. They are immortal. Cells divide a limited number of times. Cells obtained from a newborn or a fetus live longer than cells obtained from an adult, because they are capable of dividing more times. Damages over a lifetime to an older person's face are irreversible because the cells have slowed down or stopped dividing.

Genetic research has uncovered what seems to control the division of cells. Every strand of DNA in every cell of the body is capped by a string of genetic material, which apparently has no other function than to control the life of the cell. This bit of genetic code is called a telomere. Each time a cell divides, a small piece of the telomere is lost. After a certain number of divisions, the telomere is used up and this is thought to be a signal to the cell that it's time to die and make room for younger cells. In other words, telomeres act as cellular aging clocks, ticking off the number of times each cell divides before it becomes obsolete.

Cancer cells contain an enzyme called telomerase, which adds pieces of genetic code back onto the telomere after each cell division. The end result of this process is cellular immortality, i.e., the cells never get the message that it's time to die. They continue to multiply and spread, displacing healthy tissues nearby.

Cells also divide at a slower rate as we age. Our bodies are masterful self-healers. Each of our cells has repair mechanisms and self-maintenance programs running 24 hours a day. Not only are these self-protective and self-healing mechanisms efficient, but they are making and exchanging atoms within individual molecules all the time. But the repair mechanism does lose its capability as we age. Thus, *skin cells, like most other types of cells, have limited divides or life. The older the skin, the slower the divides, thus the slower the healing.*

A series of important experiments has shown how oxygen influences cellular growth and life span. It was found that oxygen is actually very bad for cell growth. Fresh sea level room air, or most of the environment we live in, contains about 20% oxygen, not the most optimal environment for cell growth. Most types of skin cells, whether in culture or healing wounds, grow best at oxygen levels similar to those carried inside the body, about 1-2% oxygen. At such low oxygen concentration, cells not only grow faster but they live longer—somewhat contradictory to common belief. We tend to think we need fresh air with more oxygen to keep our skin in great condition.

If we apply a little common sense, it is not hard to understand the results of such experiments. We all know how oxygen oxidizes metal. That is how a brown-colored copper turns green. This is how metal structures turn rusty. There are more examples in our life. When we cut vegetables and fruits, they become oxidized at the cut, forming a brown-colored layer. In fact, the free radical theory of aging believes that aging is due to oxidants combining with DNA and other body structures such as proteins to form derivatives. Over time, these free radicals degenerate the body systems.

Another simple observation is to compare people living in warm and humid climates with people in dry places. Everything else being equal (especially the amount of sun exposure), people living in warm, humid places tend to have better skin. This is because their skin is constantly covered with the sweat and oil that the body secretes as well as moisture in the air, which seal off the impact of oxygen attack. Their skin lives longer and regenerates faster if damaged. On the other hand, people living in dry places tend to have beaten-up skin. Thus, a simple basic principle for maintaining a youthful look: *Skin lives longer and heals quicker in a very low oxygen environment of less than 1-2% oxygen.*

Another major discovery in skin aging is linked to the free radical theory of aging. It is well known that in the process of consuming energy, the cells generate free radical byproducts. These are unstable oxygen molecules. Free radicals can attach themselves to other atoms and molecules, such as proteins, causing general aging. A less-known discovery is that most of the damage by free radicals is in the outer layer of the cell, called the cell plasma membrane, rather than the interior of the cell, such as cellular DNA. The free radicals are drawn to areas that have the greatest density of molecules in the outer layers. Once the cell's outer layer is damaged, it becomes inefficient at letting nutrients in and letting waste out (such as salt). As a result, the cell becomes dehydrated and looks old. *The outer layer of the cell is mostly fat. Most anti-aging facial creams are water soluble rather than fat soluble, because the conventional wisdom is that the free-radical damage occurs in the interior of the cell that is water-soluble. However, it's important to use an oil soluble anti-oxidant cream, which can penetrate into the outer layer of the skin cell.*

Sunlight is the most common cause of skin damage, but this is a very complex subject. On the one hand, most of us know that we need sunlight to get vitamin D and more importantly to absorb cosmic energy. Sunlight also gives us a tanned healthy look, a symbol of the wealth and leisure lifestyle. Corporate executives like to wear suntans, simply to demonstrate that they have a great life outside of work despite their busy schedules.

On the other hand, we all have some knowledge about how sunlight damages the skin and causes skin cancer. We often stand in line (in front of a Disney ride or movie ticket booth) watching the person in front of us with brown spots all over his shoulders, arms, face, and neck. For many, the skin is completely destroyed, despite how well they may look at a distance. Many of us believe that if we apply enough sunscreen, we'll be just fine. We will explain how this is not necessarily the case.

So what is wrong with beaten-up skin if we can exchange it for the joy of the suntan and the fun? It makes a world of difference from a longevity point of view. We want you not only to be much younger than your peer group from biological, physiological, and spiritual points of view, but also to look 20 years younger than them. Beaten-up skin on the face and neck will make you look extremely old, especially after the 40's.

By the law of limited divides, we have a little more luxury to expose more of ourselves under the sun while younger than 15 years of age. This is because we have a high ability to repair the damaged skin cells and regenerate new ones. When we get older, the damage becomes partially repairable and partially unrepairable. Therefore we acquire permanent marks.

Before we go into the scientific evidence of the impact of sunlight, let's look at how it works in nature. Most of us remember our parents urging us to go out and play in the sunshine. We grew up believing in its beneficence. Why, if it has the capacity to cause such disfigurement and even death, have humans evolved in its light?   After all, some would ask, "Isn't it true that sunlight is part of nature and we are meant to play amid nature?" This is not completely true. Animals sometimes are more spiritual, having an innate sense of nature because their minds are not complicated by the materialism that humans face. By watching them, we can understand a lot about nature, since we gradually lost the ability to connect with nature as we evolved.

Animals don't spend a lot of time under the sun by choice. They perform activities under the sun by necessity, such as searching for food, escaping from predators, playing. But they don't deliberately get a tan. In fact, on a hot day they lie down in the shade whenever possible. On the other hand, we often see humans baking themselves under direct sunlight. Animals are also protected by fur against cold and sunlight.

Let's now look at scientific studies about sunlight. Sunlight waves consist of a wide spectrum of energy. The shorter the wavelength, the more energy it carries. Life on earth can tolerate only a small portion of the wide spectrum of sunlight waves. Humans can naturally perceive (see and feel) a small portion of the light spectrum from the sun. We see the different color lights at the low spectrum; we sense the warmth of the infrared light energy. But the rest of the sun's powerful waves, like X rays or ultraviolet waves, surround us unnoticed.

Ultraviolet (UV) light waves are the most damaging to human skin. UV light also has several different wavelengths. The longest wavelengths penetrate deepest into the skin, and cause the most potential damage. When sunlight hits the skin, it is absorbed by a type of molecule called pigment melanin. Melanin is what makes our skin dark, both naturally and after sun exposure. The amount of melanin determines our natural skin color. White people have very little melanin. Melanin protects the genetic machinery of our cells by absorbing sunlight and turning the skin darker—tan. Severe sun exposure will cause a lack of sufficient protection from melanin. The lighter our natural skin color, the harder it is to protect ourselves from the sun.

Many of us are exposed not only to direct sunlight, but also to various forms of UV lights. For example, the so-called "black lights" or UV lamps are used to kill bacteria in the food processing industry. We also treat acne under UV lights. Tanning beds employ UV light to produce an artificial tan.

There are several subspectrums within UV light— UVA, UVB, UVC. UVA has the longest wavelength of the three. UVC is normally filtered out entirely by the earth's atmosphere, so the main impact on us is UVA and UVB.

Many people believe that UVA is safe. For example, tanning bed operators use UVA light and claim it does not damage the skin. Most sunscreens are rated by SPF numbers that refer only to the effect of UVB radiation because UVA is assumed to be safe.

The fact is that both UVA and UVB are damaging. Thus, using artificial UVA tanning light or sunscreens may not protect us from skin damage.

UVB radiation has long been considered the root cause of sunburn. Exposure to UVB causes a burning sensation quickly and leaves an initial reddish cast. Delayed tanning occurs several days after the initial exposure as a result of increased activity or increased production of melanin stimulated by the UVB exposure.

UVA, on the other hand, does not burn the skin directly. But it does produce an immediate tan. The majority of solar ultraviolet radiation that reaches the earth's surface is UVA. This is why the conventional wisdom claims that UVA is safe. Unfortunately, it is becoming increasingly clear that no UV exposure is safe. UVA can penetrate deep into the skin, causing damage to DNA and leading to wrinkling, spotting, and skin cancers we wrongly attribute to normal aging. UVA also injures blood vessels, causing the broken capillaries often seen on the nose and cheeks of sun-damaged individuals. UVA can also burn the eyes, resulting in cataracts over time.

Eventually a suntan recedes, giving the impression that any damage done is gone forever. But the damage is a lot deeper. As we age, our systems simply cannot repair or replace all the damaged cells deep below the surface of the skin. The accumulation of this damage accelerates aging. Thus, *both UVA and UVB exposure creates significant skin damage. There is no safe protection even to UVA exposure only.*

Not only is skin damaged from UV light due to insufficient melanin protection, but sunlight intensifies the oxidation process. As we discussed earlier, skin cells live best in a moist, low oxygen concentration environment. Sunlight bakes out the natural and applied oil of the skin and dries up skin moisture. Think of frying an egg in an oiled pan. The heat will dry up the oil and fry the egg. Similarly, we often see older people on the beach with their skin hanging like dried paper folds, baking in the sun oven. Their skin has been baked dry and oxidized to the maximum. *Long-term UV exposure intensifies skin oxidation.*

Chinese medicine believes the lung meridian controls all respiratory functions. Skin is considered an organ belonging to the lung meridian system. Thus the lung meridian controls the health of the skin. The skin, or surface layer of the body, is particularly dependent on nourishment provided by the lung in the form of wei chi (energy flowing through energy meridians between skin and flesh) and body fluid. At the same time, the skin assists the lung function. The sweat pore is known in Chinese medicine as the "portal of energy"; the opening and closing of these pores are governed by wei chi, which in turn is dependent on the lung's dispersing function. The skin thus assists in dispersing wei chi and in regulating respiration. *For healthy skin, the lung meridian must be balanced and energized.*

A much-overlooked cause of skin aging is the fast and feast cycle. In today's industrialized society, there is seldom a lack of food and nutrition. Food as a necessity becomes less important than food as part of the enjoyment of life. Going to an upscale restaurant, having a drink, partying, meeting interesting people, negotiating business deals—all are conducted in a food setting. Thus we are accustomed to eating more than we need.

We, as a society, have become fat. As a result, many people periodically go on diets. These weight loss programs range from strict fasting on fruit juice only to powdered supplements. Most of the time, we lose a few pounds and quickly gain them back when we return to a normal routine. Seldom are people willing to live on such programs forever and completely change the lifestyle which got them into obesity in the first place. As a result, they go through fast and feast cycles, becoming fat, then thin, then fat again. As we age, our skin gradually loses elasticity. It does not shrink automatically when we reduce in size. Therefore our skin hangs in many folds as the fat is lost, another root cause of why we look older than we should. *Maintain the same adult weight throughout your lifetime to minimize the impact of lost skin elasticity in aging.*

THE HEALTH OF BONES

There are two main types of bone problems as we age. First, the bones are worn and damaged through lifelong hard work and exercise, the famous osteoarthritis: the swelling and stiffening of the weight-bearing joints of the body. Many bone surgeries are due to damage from playing sports when young. Second, bone problems arise from loss of calcium and other vital essence, resulting in osteoporosis, the thinning bone condition that causes humped backs and fractures of the hip and spine.

Osteoarthritis results when the spongy cartilage, or gristle, of the joints grinds away, leaving joint bones raw and unpadded. Again, exercises can be a two-edged sword. Certain forms of strenuous exercise may make us prone to arthritis, particularly weight lifting, push-ups, football, and baseball. Light to moderate exercise, such as jogging, biking, swimming, and walking can actually help prevent arthritis by keeping the bones, ligaments, and cartilage in good working order.

The back, neck, hips, and knees are prone to arthritis, especially after a lifetime of sports injury, trauma, or even just bad posture. Ballet dancers tend to develop arthritis in their feet; tennis players tend to get it in their elbows and joggers in their knees. Obesity has been linked with arthritis, too, from joints having to bear excess weight. Computer engineers tend to be constantly in one posture, creating strain on the lower back.

Unlike muscles, joints register wounds at a much younger age. A twisted ankle at age 13 during a basketball game will likely be twisted in the same place many times during life. Even if we are young, the damage never goes away completely. It heals but is always weaker than the original. *Bone can never recover to its pre-injured strength. Avoid unnecessary strenuous exercises.*

Osteoporosis is usually defined as enough bone loss to be diagnosed on an X ray or to have caused at least one fracture. When bone loss shows up in X ray, it has lost at least 30% of bone mass. As we age, calcium in bones starts to diffuse out of the bone into the blood stream. The bone becomes loose and less dense. Nutritionists advise taking plenty of calcium supplements to compensate for the loss. However, even with sufficient calcium, the body may be very inefficient in metabolizing the calcium, and the bones can be inefficient in absorbing it. A more fundamental path to bone health is maintaining balanced and high energy kidney meridians .

Traditional Chinese medicine believes that the vital essence stored by the kidneys forms bone marrow. The bones, in turn, grow strong when properly nourished by the marrow. Marrow is of two types: bone marrow and the spinal marrow that permeates the brain. Chinese medicine asserts that the brain is formed of marrow and hence calls it the "reservoir of marrow." Since marrow is formed out of vital essence from the kidneys, the brain is closely connected with the kidneys. When the kidney meridian is healthy, nutrients and minerals are metabolized and bone marrow is full of bone-nourishing nutrients such as calcium. *For healthy bones and joints, the kidney meridian must be balanced and highly energized.*

APPLYING THE PROTOCOL

The *PingLongevity* protocol for preserving the body's mechanical system is very simple:
- Avoid strenuous exercise after age 25

- Train muscles when young (before age 20)
- Engage in light movement, such as swimming, tai chi, walking, etc.
- Use oil-soluble anti-oxidant facial creams, followed by an oil which seals oxygen the most to the face and neck
- Allow no direct sun exposure to facial skin and neck
- Avoid large weight loss and gain
- Take herbal supplements for lung, kidney, and spleen meridian energy balance

If we enjoy sports activities, we can still try to reduce strenuous sports as we age because we have less ability to recover from injuries. You can reduce and stop the type of boring exercises done simply for weight control. Build muscles early in life. Use other *PingLongevity* protocols to control weight through food therapy rather than through eat and burn methods.

Mind and body movement is the best exercise of all. It combines spirit and body. It channels physical strength as well as subtle energy throughout the body. Tai chi is the best of such forms. Note that it is counterintuitive to some of the modern methods, where body and mind are forcefully pulling apart, such as walking a treadmill while watching TV or jogging while listening to the radio.

What are the best oxygen seals for the face and neck? The more oil-based the sealer, the better it is. There is a fad of applying nutrients to the face, and many new creams and lotions have been developed. But their effects are only temporary. The only magic solution is to seal oxygen and nourish the lungs. Therefore, a simple, inexpensive thick pure oil is the most effective. Some examples of the best oils are pure emu oil, lanolin, and non-petroleum jelly. What are the best anti-oxidants? The most powerful anti-oxidants are *oil soluble* vitamin C, alpha lipoic acid, and alpha hydroxy and beta hydroxy acids.

How can we avoid the enjoyment of the beautiful sun? We can do most outdoor activities by taking a few precautions. Wear hats, long-sleeve shirts and pants under heavy sunlight. Swim in late afternoon or early morning. A cloudy day is the best for bare-headed outdoor activities. For those who really like a heavy tan, try creams that give a tan color rather than exposing your skin to the UV light.

If there is a will, we can find a way both to enjoy nature and avoid direct sunlight that damages our skin. We should not compromise our quality of life. In fact, we enhance it through the vibrant youth we can achieve.

Follow our other protocols to keep weight constant throughout your life, the same weight when you were 18-22 years old. That is your own genetically optimal weight. Forget about the recommended weight, which is other people's average and has nothing to do with your own genetic inheritance.

Follow the protocols presented in the next chapter for herbal balancing of lung, spleen, and kidney meridians to achieve skin, muscle, and bone health.

CHAPTER 6

FOURTH PROTOCOL: BALANCE ENERGY MERIDIANS

I sat by the fireplace in Sara's home today, taking part in a discussion group that included a few MDs, a couple of acupuncturists, three herbalists, and the manager of a health-care network.

"I am frustrated," said Mike, one of the MDs. "I see patients taking too many drugs yet can't help prescribing more for them. It may start with anti-inflammatory drugs for joint and muscle pain, but soon their stomachs hurt due to the side effects. So I have to put them on a stomach pill. Often they become depressed from the pain. So they have to take an antidepressant or mood medicine. Their sleep is disturbed and they use sleeping pills. Some of these patients take medication ten times a day. It's a vicious cycle. They must take medicine. We prescribe it. Then comes the side effects, and they take more drugs. According to a new statistics cited by *USA Today*, January 31, 2001 issue, more than 44% of Americans take prescription drugs daily. Approximately 9% take more than 5 prescription drugs daily."

Sally, a nutritionist, joined in, "I know what you're talking about. I give out Vitamins A, B, C, D, E, and lots more. New nutrients and supplements that the body requires are discovered every day. I don't want them to miss any. Patients complain, but what can I do? Every single one of these nutrients and supplements is good for them. So they take 30-50 capsules a day."

"I am like you," said Jim, the herbalist. "They come to me for natural healing. Most are tired of conventional medicine and many drugs. They have multiple problems: headaches, high blood pressure, high cholesterol, joint pain, ringing ears. I have hundreds of different formulas suitable for each of these symptoms. I usually choose a good formula which can treat a couple of them, and continue to choose other formulas for other symptoms. In the end, it amounts to a lot. Besides, I have to tell them, 'Don't drop the medicines prescribed by your MD. When you feel better, talk to your doctor. He may take you off the medicine.' I feel sorry for these people. They are taking too many things."

"I used to do the same," I said, "carrying hundreds of different formulas in my office. But now I have just eight, and things are much better. These eight fundamental formulas can deal with almost every disease by rebalancing the major organ energy systems. A patient may have multiple symptoms. But according to traditional Chinese medicine, the symptoms are only signals that tell you one of the major organ systems is under stress or out of balance. If you treat the symptoms, you are only helping part of the body, instead of treating the major root causes. You need to look at a combination of symptoms to find out what is the cause of those symptoms deep inside the body."

"Tell us how it works, Ping," said one of the doctors in the group.

"I treated a patient with low back pain. After a few sessions of taking kidney support herbs, his pain was completely eased. In his last visit, he asked, 'Ping, what did you do to me? I had ear ringing for years and couldn't find relief. I never told you about it because other doctors hadn't helped, and I thought you probably couldn't treat it either. I came to get my back better, but now my back is fine and my ears stopped ringing too.'

"I had been trying to strengthen his internal kidney meridian. When the kidneys are strong, all kidney-related symptoms go away. Ear ringing and low back pain are both related to kidney energy. So taking the kidney support herbs balanced the energy. This is why both symptoms are gone, even though we did not specifically treat the ear ringing.

"Another example was a lady with arthritis. I gave her bone and joint formula. After a few weeks, she told me, 'This herb has something to do with my kidney.' I asked why. She said, 'I used to go to the bathroom every two hours at night, and had a very thin and slow stream of urine. After taking these herbs, my joints are better and so is the urination. I only get up once a night and have a good strong stream of urine, just like before.'

"Now think about it. If all our organ energy systems are strong and balanced, all symptoms should go away. We are protected from virus and bacteria. Even someone who doesn't have symptoms can still use the herbs for anti-aging so their systems will stay in balance."

To my delight, the others in the room agreed with me and wondered how to get the word out that balancing the fundamental organ energy systems can give us an energy system which heals itself of all symptoms and diseases and keeps us young for a long time.

Ping's Diary

All of us have three major planes of being: the physical plane, the energy plane, and the spiritual plane. They range from lower to higher energy frequencies of the universe.

The first three protocols work on the physical plane. This protocol is devoted to the energy plane. After practicing the first three, our blood is healthily "thin" with less sugar, less fat, less pressure and vibrantly flows throughout the body. In this protocol, we will talk about how to get chi balanced and flowing unobstructively through the body meridians (energy channels).

Like blood, chi (energy) is the sustaining force of every part of us. It flows invisibly through energy channels, called meridians in traditional Chinese medicine. These meridians are not physically seen and don't correspond to anything in anatomy. However, plenty of modern scientific research has proven that such higher subtle energy exists. Chi can be partially measured and has some property of electromagnetic energy. Meridians are also proven to be along low electrical resistant points in the body, the so-called acupuncture points.

In the language of the energy universe already described, we know this energy is of higher frequency—a frequency beyond current technology measurement. Still, these are life-sustaining forces just like blood. Think about stirring a cup of milk using a stick. The round motion of the stick creates a curvature of the milk surface inside the cup. The edge of the milk surface is higher and the middle sinks down. This surface shape needs to be sustained by the energy transmitted from the stick. If the energy becomes weaker, the shape of the surface becomes flatter. If the energy of the stirring falls to zero, the surface flattens. There is more life if the curvature is higher.

Once the energy is balanced and vibrant, the body is free from all diseases and lives with maximum youth. This is exactly the principle of acupuncture and herbal medicine. When energy is blocked, or unbalanced, it flows through the meridians in an unbalanced way. Acupuncture needles inserted at energy points along meridians cause the meridian to rebalance its stagnated energy flow due to the stimulation and sometimes the energy transmission from the acupuncturist's hands. We use acupuncture when we are sick. In order to have vibrant health, we want to open and balance our meridians automatically every minute throughout the whole body before we are sick.

This protocol will present ways, through both herbs and chi-gong, to insert many invisible "acupuncture needles" into ourselves constantly to assure that all meridians are balanced.

It is interesting to note the ancient Greek definition of aging: Aging is a disease that results from an imbalance in the "four humours" (blood, phlegm, yellow bile, and black bile).

From the modern medical point of view, imbalance can at least be characterized in the physical plane. For example, disease arises when enzyme activities are imbalanced. There are too many enzyme activities that induce unwanted results, such as stimulating cancer growth; and there are too few enzyme activities that inhibit the wanted results, such as immune response. Thus, imbalance can be partially explained by the imbalance of enzyme activities. As a result of enzyme imbalance, hormones and other body systems become imbalanced. However, the imbalance from the modern medical point of view is not complete. It does not include the higher energy and spiritual planes.

There are many reasons meridians get closed, blocked, and unbalanced. The environment puts us through many emergency responses that necessarily kick us off balance. When we face a stressful situation, our systems automatically release hormones to instruct the body to shut down normal body processes, such as digestion, and focus all energy on the situation at hand (you can feel your heart pump faster instantly). When we catch a cold, our body has to declare a state of emergency (high fever, for instance) to deal with the situation. When our normal perfect equilibrium is off balance, we don't return exactly to the same place—usually far from it. We settle down at a new energy place, which is all unbalanced. Thus the body starts to work suboptimally, and the situation is made worse by modern materialism. An increased craving for money, fame, and power has increased formerly "accepted standards," thus deliberately becoming "un-natural" to our original nature. We turn desire, such as sex, into indulgence. We become the hardest working species on earth. As a result, there is a heightened trend toward unbalanced energy meridians.

There are two methods of balancing our energy systems: (1) the herbal method, which uses a system of herbs to balance the body's energy meridians; and (2) chi-gong. *Chi* in Chinese means "of energy"; *gong* means "work." So chi-gong is the work to balance and direct the flow of chi through the meridians. The second method is more advanced and more difficult to learn. However, it is a vastly rewarding way because the body can now balance more naturally with its own force. Both methods will be used in our longevity protocols.

HERBAL BALANCING OF ENERGY

Chinese medicine has the longest undisturbed history of compiling knowledge, from the shamans of ancient folk lore to modern-day physicians and scientists, spanning 5,000 years of wisdom that integrates the art with the science of healing.

Every disease is considered a result of imbalance of yin and yang of meridians and major organs. There are more than 3,000 Chinese herbs and thousands of combination formulas developed in the 5,000 years of Chinese medicine. These are time-proven formulas noted in Chinese medicine classics. However, application of these many formulas is complex. Each formula is used to compensate or cool down a particular symptom of disease. It becomes more of an art than a repeatable science.

Traditional Chinese doctors, the artists, use their own combinations of herbs and their own method of acupuncture to treat patients. Many of the formulas are passed down from generation to generation; only male members of the family have the privilege of inheriting the secrecy. Likewise, acupuncture can be applied to so many points and combinations of points, depending on the acupuncturist. The effectiveness of acupuncture is also dependent on the chi (energy) through the hands of the healers. That explains why the variation of effectiveness of herbal formulas and acupuncture treatment is so large among alternative doctors. It is like oil paintings. Certain artists can make a tremendous impact on the art form.

Western medicine is different. Based on symptoms, doctors order a battery of tests (blood work, X rays, CT, urine test, etc.) to diagnose patients. Once results show positive, a prescribed set of medicine/treatment (not invented by the doctors, but provided by a few large pharmaceutical companies and approved by the government regulatory agencies) is administrated (drugs, chemotherapy). Western medicine is more than an art form.

The goal for those who want good health is to combine the best of traditional Chinese medicine with the Western variety, to make this available to all people, and to reduce the variations of quality provided by practitioners. This not only requires standardization in formulas but also simplicity in application, one of the hurdles preventing traditional Chinese medicine from maximum effectiveness for all.

In order to develop a much more simplified herbal protocol for health and longevity, let's first discuss some very basic concepts in traditional Chinese medicine.

YIN-YANG PRINCIPLE

Traditional Chinese medicine is based mainly on the yin-yang principle, the five-element theory, and the body's energy meridian systems.

Yin and yang are two opposite poles. Without yin, there is no yang. They must co-exist to make a whole. Examples are cold and hot, low and high, wet and dry, earth and heaven, north and south. When yin and yang are not equal, the equilibrium is broken. In human health, yin mostly refers to essence or substance: blood, semen, hormones, saliva, enzymes, etc. Yang refers to energy (chi) to sustain the body's activities. For example, heart is yang in transferring blood and blood is yin. The heart energy to transport blood and the availability of blood form the yin and yang aspect of the heart meridian system. If heart energy is low, the transportation lacks vitality. If blood is lacking, the body cannot be nourished. To treat heart meridian-related diseases, we must first identify if it is a yang deficiency or a yin deficiency. Then we use herbs that can treat the corresponding deficiency to heal the body.

In general, there are four types of yin and yang imbalance: too strong yin, which impairs yang; too strong yang, which overconsumes yin; deficiency in yin; and deficiency in yang. In the ancient classic *Plain Questions*, it was said that "a deficiency of yang brings on exterior cold, while a deficiency of yin leads to interior heat. A preponderance of yang leads to exterior heat, while a preponderance of yin leads to interior cold." Using the heart example, when yang is deficient (e.g., lack of heart energy), the symptom is a pale face, a thin, white-coated tongue, depression, etc. This is because the circulation of blood is not strong.

FIVE-ELEMENT THEORY

The concept of the five-element theory was developed several thousand years ago. The ancient Chinese came up with the system to describe the relationships and changes in nature. They used five phenomena of earth and heaven to symbolize and provide analogies for all things in the universe. The medical application of the five-element theory is only one application.

These five phenomena are earth, water, metal, wood, and fire. The relationship is that earth promotes metal (think about gold formed in the earth); metal promotes water; water promotes wood; wood promotes fire; and fire promotes earth (by burning down things to return to the earth). You can see the cycle that makes nature a self-sustaining loop. The five elements also overcome each other. Water overcomes fire, fire overcomes metal, metal overcomes wood, wood overcomes earth (when roots cut into earth), and earth overcomes water (by blocking water). The relationship is illustrated below.

Five Elements Relationship

→ Promoting relationship
⋯⋯⋯⋯⋯→ Overcoming relationship

We can apply the five-element theory to many natural phenomena. Its application provides another cornerstone besides yin-yang in traditional Chinese medicine. The human body is classified by five large energy meridian systems: the heart, lung, spleen, liver, and kidney. These are not mere organs in the conventional medical sense but are systems that function as organs as well as energy systems.

For example, from a mechanical view of modern medicine, the spleen is considered part of the lymphatic system. The spleen filters blood and produces antibodies—the white cells. It is also considered somewhat noncritical. Often you hear about surgical removal of a spleen due to liver disease or injury in an auto accident. Nevertheless, the spleen system is considered extremely important in traditional Chinese medicine. The spleen system connects to the stomach, governing transportation and transformation of food, and dominates muscles and limbs. An impaired spleen function results in mental turmoil, often marked by irritability, poor memory, and flaccid limbs. It manifests itself in the mouth (appetite, taste) and lips (pale, swollen).

These five main energy systems are put in the language of five elements in order to study the interrelationship: fire is associated with heart, earth with spleen, kidney with water, lung with metal, and liver with wood. These are not random associations but are based on the interrelationship of these meridian systems. It is a demonstration that traditional Chinese medicine thinks of the human body as a whole. When a lung is in trouble, unlike conventional medicine that treats lung (metal), traditional Chinese medicine looks also into spleen because spleen is earth, which promotes metal. It also looks into the heart (fire) because fire overcomes metal. Too strong a heart energy or too weak a spleen function will weaken lung energy. When the body is considered interrelated in the energy sense, rather than an interlink of mechanical parts, it becomes very complex.

Another example of the difference between traditional Chinese medicine and modern medicine is shown in the treatment of osteoporosis, a disease in which calcium is lost from the bones, resulting in reduced bone density. The modern medicine treatment is to take dietary supplements of Vitamin D and calcium and hope the bones will absorb more supplements. Recent progress also makes bone replacement possible. On the other hand, traditional Chinese medicine considers bone problems a kidney deficiency.

Kidney filters blood, gets rid of waste and toxins, and reabsorbs nutrients and minerals, including calcium and magnesium. If the kidney system is healthy, and enough calcium and magnesium are in the diet, kidneys can reabsorb sufficient calcium and magnesium into the body. Vitamin D is also converted to its active form of D3 in the kidney system. With Vitamin D, calcium and magnesium can be absorbed into the bones. Thus, your body can restore your bone health through strengthening your kidney function. Since we are not growing taller, our requirement for large doses of calcium is not very high. In general, it is not that we don't have enough calcium in our diet; it is our weakened kidney function after middle age. Thus we must treat the root cause of the bone disease and consider the body as a whole system instead of an assembly of mechanical parts.

THE MERIDIAN SYSTEMS

There is a simple way to practice traditional Chinese medicine. The breakthrough is based on yin-yang and the five-element theory. The new method treats the fundamental imbalance and weakness of the energy meridian systems rather than the specific diseases. It claims that once the fundamental system is back to optimal condition, diseases disappear and can be prevented. The theory focuses on the five fundamental energy meridian systems:

heart, lung, liver, kidney, spleen. Each of these five systems, when imbalanced, is either too low in yin and thus too high in yang, or vice versa. We need only eight herbal formulas to address the root causes of diseases. This is a major breakthrough because eight fundamental formulas, instead of thousands, can be used to regenerate the body to its optimal balance.

To further specify the eight formulas, we use a heart formula to treat heart yin imbalance (due to insufficient supply of heart essence, i.e., blood to the heart); a lung yin formula to treat yin deficiency (due to inability to carry sufficient oxygen through the lung); a cleansing formula to calm overabundance of heart or lung energy (yang disease); a kidney yin formula to treat yin deficiency (due to insufficient kidney essence, such as hormones, bone marrow, spinal fluid, joint fluid, semen, etc.); a kidney yang formula to treat yang deficiency (energy or chi); a liver yin formula to treat liver yin deficiency (due to insufficient production of blood); a liver yang formula to treat the overabundance of yang (due to overactive liver functions); a spleen yang formula to treat spleen yang deficiency (due to insufficient spleen energy or chi). Therefore, a total of eight formulas can help balance the body's five major organ meridian systems. Once the systems are balanced, the body can heal itself.

The application is also very simple. Traditional Chinese medicine uses several diagnostic methods. One is pulse taking, when a doctor takes a patient's pulse to figure out the internal issues of the body. The second method is observance. Traditional Chinese medicine believes that all internal diseases and energy imbalance are pictured in the appearance of the body. For example, eyes are associated with liver. Unclear white of the eye gives clues about liver condition. Bones and ears are associated with the kidney. Bone and ear problems point to a kidney yin-yang imbalance. Through observation, good traditional Chinese medicine doctors can not only pinpoint the root causes of diseases accurately, but also detect issues far in advance of modern medical equipment. This is because observation at the subtle energy level is always in advance of the physical level. Thus, associated with the eight herbal formulas are eight sets of symptoms to point out the areas of energy imbalance and deficiency.

Now we can see the beauty of the new theory: eight formulas and eight sets of symptoms for diagnosis instead of thousands. Today, we are bombarded with hundreds of different types of vitamins, herbs, and supplements, each one targeted to treat certain symptoms. As we become more health conscious, we want to take them all. But should we? How useful are they? The answer is, we must get back to the fundamentals, and there are only a handful which are truly needed for vibrant health.

There is a major difference between conventional medicine and traditional Chinese medicine. Say you have a blood chemistry test. The results come back as a bacteria infection. So you take antibiotics, which kill bacteria. But you have not done anything to help the body fundamentally by asking questions: Why did I so easily contract the bacteria? Why not others? Is there a deeper root cause? Will I get it again? Although the bacteria is dead, the job is not done. In traditional Chinese medicine, it is more important to get the body back to its optimal balance so you will not get infections so easily next time. We all have experienced a cold that dragged on for a long time, and after it was over we soon caught another one. Other people who seem resistant to colds have a much more balanced system deep inside the body.

LISTENING TO OUR BODIES

Evaluating the condition of our health and the balance of our energy systems based on observation of our own symptoms is a very important concept. We believe this can benefit everyone.

Although we conventionally trust our doctors for their understanding of scientific research in medicine, we are the first to experience our body's symptoms. We can *feel* them better than anyone else can see them. When the body speaks, there is something happening. By learning how to interpret the messages (symptoms), we not only listen to our body but also understand its language. Not everyone can become a doctor. But we should not be blind either. If we are, we lose a lot of valuable early information that our body is trying to relate to us. Nobody outside of us can get that information as well as we can ourselves. After all, we care more about ourselves, more than our doctors or neighbors do.

Many times, symptoms are early signs of system imbalance. Symptoms are the daily reports our soldiers in the body relate to us through our senses and observations. Diseases in their infancy may or may not develop into severe illness. Most of the time, the early symptoms are not associated with the definition of disease in the context of modern medicine. Frequently, we go to a doctor telling him about our pain or inability to sleep well. The doctor tells us that nothing is wrong or that he can do nothing. This is because the symptoms have not developed into medically defined "diseases" yet.

However, in the sense of preventative medicine, we know there must be some small imbalance happening. We must correct it. If not, the small imbalance will mushroom into larger ones. If we don't take the reports from the soldiers guarding our bodies, we will later find out that the invaders have become too strong for us to throw out. We must deal with these early symptoms ourselves. We need to inspect ourselves, every day.

Traditional Chinese medicine uses several diagnostic methods, such as to look, listen, ask questions, feel the pulse, check body temperature. Even with today's modern medicine, these methods are still important. How we feel and look is more important than simply what test results show. Many times people who have reported symptoms to doctors and gone through batteries of tests that showed only negative results finally wound up seeing a psychologist, thinking maybe their mind was wrong. We have seen so many patients who have symptoms such as pain, but tests show nothing abnormal. But this pain is accompanied by symptoms that do mean something in the Chinese medicine method. A patient may have red, irritated eyes, or a red or pale coating on the tongue, or a weak or a thin, tight pulse. The pain is due to meridian blockage and organ imbalance and is not bad enough to have tests show abnormal results. But if left untreated, it *will* develop into serious disease.

Let's talk in more detail about observation. A person's face is a very good place to read internal conditions. A pale face indicates anemia or heart energy deficiency. A rusty, dark face color could be kidney energy imbalance. Bags or dark circles under and around the eyes may come from liver imbalance. Acne, pimples, or rashes may be the sign of lung disease. Yellow color may be due to liver or spleen imbalance. A blue purplish face or lips may be the stagnation of heart blood.

Eyes are very important too. They are associated with the liver. Red swelling or yellow sclera suggests liver imbalance. Nose discharge, running nose, and red nose all suggest lung imbalance. Ear is associated with kidney. Dry withered auricles or a burnt black color suggest the kidney is under stress. Gum redness and swelling could be related to stomach digestion. It is also important to observe the tongue, which is a storehouse for diagnosis information. In general, over-red, over-pale, dryness, or cracking in the middle of the tongue suggests some form of imbalance of different body systems. Similarly, we can diagnose based on listening and smelling. Is your own talking voice strong or weak? Is your breath rough or light? Do bad odors emanate from the body, for example, bad breath or smelly urine?

We know that eyes are related to liver, ears to kidney, nose to lung, lips to spleen, and tongue to heart. We also know that emotions are related to our energy systems. Anger hurts the liver system, sadness impairs the lung, overjoy shocks the heart, fear stresses the kidney, and overthinking hurts the spleen.

When the kidney is imbalanced, our soldiers signal a dis-function. The ear is simply one of our kidney signals. If we don't consider the body as an interconnected, whole system, we may see it isolated by different parts. We may have to see heart specialists, then come back to see a lung specialist, then go to a psychologist for counseling, then see a bone specialist and arthritis specialist, with each doctor seeing a part of us. Our condition could start with rheumatic fever, later develop into heart murmur, years later de-velop into heart failure, kidney failure, and water in the lung. Thus one small symptom can develop into serious life-threatening dis-eases. This is exactly why we want to use the eight fundamental formulas.

A group of symptoms seemingly unrelated may actually come from the same root cause. One may feel dryness and redness in the eyes, irritability and anger, headaches, weariness, high cho-lesterol and blood pressure. All these symptoms can be associated with the yin and yang imbalance of the liver. If we treat the root cause of the imbalance, all symptoms will disappear. However, if we treat each symptom separately—painkiller for headache, eye drops, physical therapy for back pain, pills for high blood pres-sure—each medicine will do its job to suppress the symptom one by one. Now we as the commanders have shut up our soldiers who tried to report the enemy invaders. We completely disabled the signals! The enemy is already in our castle; the true root cause (an imbalance in our liver) is growing stronger and stronger. Finally, it becomes too late for us to do anything but surrender.

Many recent discoveries confirm the holistic approach of traditional Chinese medicine. For example, in her book *The Fat*

Flush Plan, nutritionist Ann Louise Gittleman presents a breakthrough diet plan that focuses on cleansing of toxins in the liver—a system fundamental to metabolic efficiency. She writes, "Your liver is a workhorse that can even regenerate its own damaged cells. However, it is not invincible. When it lacks essential nutrients or when it is overwhelmed by toxins, it no longer performs as it should. Hormone imbalances may develop. Fat may accumulate in the liver and then just under the skin or in other organs. Toxins build up and get into your bloodstream." Among the signs of a toxic liver she names are

> Weight gain, especially around the abdomen
> Cellulite
> Abdominal bloating
> Indigestion
> High blood pressure
> Elevated cholesterol
> Fatigue
> Mood swings
> Depression
> Skin rashes"[*]

In summary, *Eight Fundamental Formulas* is a breakthrough system, which uses eight formulas to balance the yin and yang aspects of the five major organ meridians: lung, heart, liver, kidney, and spleen. Each system is associated with a set of symptoms. A set of *Eight Fundamental Tests* can identify the imbalance easily.   Application of eight rather than thousands of formulas keeps the whole body's systems in perfect balance. A balanced system can effectively heal itself.

Another breakthrough in this protocol comes from the understanding in Chinese medicine that the human body forms a mi-

---

[*] *The Fat Flush Plan*, Ann Louise Gittleman, McGraw-Hill, 2002.

crocosm, which is connected to the macrocosm of the universe. Human energy systems have peak and weak timings associated with the periodic energy field of the universe. Like Western medicine, which acknowledges that some bodily functions (such as growth hormones) peak at different times of the day, Chinese medicine believes that each body meridian goes through energy cycles every day. For example, the liver meridian reaches maximum energy between 11 p.m. and 1 a.m. Taking the meridian-balancing herbs at this time maximizes their effectiveness. Thus, each of the eight fundamental formulas is taken at a specific time of day to maximize their effect.

Chinese medicine believes the human body rejuvenates itself every 100 days. Thus, the meridian balance formulas should be taken for 100 days to re-baseline the whole body. Doctors of Western medicine believe that biological cells of the human body rejuvenate every three months. Therefore, the ancient Chinese theory has common ground with modern medical science.

SELF-TESTING FOR THE EIGHT FORMULAS

One application of the *Eight Fundamental Formulas* comes from the study of the protocols created by top medical scientists and herbalists in China. These formulas are the result of a study of China's 5,000-year-old culture and selections of prescriptions provided by classics on medicine and health. This principle of using the formulas and their associated symptom tests is summarized as follows. All these formulas are time proven and commercially available in the United States and around the world through traditional Chinese herbal stores.

Liver One Formula (also known as Xiao Cai Hu Tang Wan)

According to traditional Chinese medicine, the liver meridian controls the storage and regulation of blood and vessels. When blood is insufficient, emotion and depression occur. Liver is associated with the tendons and blood vessels. Liver manifests itself in eyes and nails. Liver One deals with liver yin deficiency: not enough blood essence to support the tendons and bones, so symptoms such as weakness of knees and/or blurred and impaired vision occur.

Self-Testing Symptoms:

Pale complexion	Hair loss
Dark circles under the eyes	Feeling sleepy all the time
Anemia	Fatigue and dizziness
Scanty menstrual period	Spasm, convulsion in tendons,,
Blurred vision	muscles
Dry eyes	Numb, weak limbs
Ophthalmologic problems	Pale, dry, brittle nails
	Depression, easily emotional

Liver Two Formula (also known as Long Dan Xie Gan Wan)

According to traditional Chinese medicine, Liver Two deals with liver yang overacting symptoms. When liver yang is overacting, anger and restlessness occur. Liver Two is associated with blood vessels and gallbladder problems as well as the detoxification of alcohol, medication, etc. Liver manifests itself in the eyes and nails.

Self-Testing Symptoms:

Redness, swelling in eyes	Weak liver function
Burning sensation of eyes	Varicose veins
Bags under the eyes	Bloating or full feeling in
Trigeminal neuralgia	chest

Migraine headache	Tenderness below the ribs
Menstrual period headache	Cholesterol above normal
Blood pressure above normal	Difficult to concentrate
Irritable, easy to get angry	Child attention deficiency

Kidney One Formula (also known as Jin Kui Shen Qi Wan)
       According to traditional Chinese medicine, the kidney me-ridian dominates human reproduction and development and water metabolism, produces marrow to fill the brain, and dominates bones. It relates to the emotions of fear and determination. It manifests itself in tooth, ear, hair, genitals, and the anus. Kidney One is associated with the yang aspect of the kidney meridian.

Self-Testing Symptoms:

Cold hands or feet	Low back pain and ache
Incontinence or frequent urination	Early menopause
Weak libido, impotence	Fear, tension, and stress
Seminal emission, premature ejaculation, infertility	Dream-disturbed sleep
Edema and swelling of legs	Shortness of breath & tiredness
Easy to catch cold, which can turn into asthma	Urinary tract, prostate problems
	Low immune system

Kidney Two Formula (also known as Liu Wei Di Huang Wan)
       According to traditional Chinese medicine, the kidney me-ridian dominates human reproduction and development and water metabolism, produces marrow to fill the brain, and dominates bone. It relates to the emotion of fears and determination. It mani-fests itself in tooth, ear, hair, genitals, and the anus. Kidney Two deals with the yin aspect of the kidney meridian. Kidney Two is

associated with the balance of hormones (e.g., menopause, night sweats, internal heat).

Self-Testing Symptoms:

Night or afternoon sweating	Anxiety, nervousness
Heat/burning in hands, feet	Decreased memory
Sweaty palms	Loose teeth
Canker sore, tongue soreness	Low back, waist soreness &
Red flush/rash over face	weakness
Burning and scanty urine	Joint and bone weakness
Hair loss or gray early	Ear ringing or hearing loss
Internal heat, desire cold	Insomnia
fluids	

Heart Formula (also known as Sheng Mai San)

     According to traditional Chinese medicine, the heart meridian governs blood and chi (energy). Blood flows through this meridian under the power of heart chi. If a person is full of vigor, blood circulates smoothly to transport nutrients to all parts of the body. The heart controls mental activities. Mental disorder arises when the heart is injured. The condition of the heart meridian manifests itself in the tongue.

Self-Testing Symptoms:

Short of breath, less energy	Shallow voice, no energy
Pale or purple tongue	when speaking
Pale face	Having appetite with no taste
Mental tiredness, easy to	Spontaneous perspiration
sigh/despair	Restless mind, insufficient
Irregular heart beat,	sleep, multiple dreams
palpitation	Easy to forget, memory loss

Spleen Formula (also known as Bu Zhong Yi Qi Wan)
According to traditional Chinese medicine, the spleen meridian connects to the stomach, governs transportation and transformation of food, and dominates muscles and limbs. An impaired spleen function results in poor digestion and absorption of nutrients. It manifests itself in the mouth (appetite, taste) and lips (pale, swollen).

Self-Testing Symptoms:

Poor digestion and absorption	Physical/mental tiredness
Reduced appetite	Pale lips and tongue
Morning loose stools, diarrhea	Heavy menstrual bleeding
Abdominal distension, heavy sensation	Muscle pain and weakness
Leaky gut	Teeth marks on the edge of tongue

Lung Formula (also known as Yang Yin Qing Fei Wan)
According to traditional Chinese medicine, the lung formula deals with lung yin deficiency. The lung meridian dominates the chi of the whole body, controls respiration, nourishes skin and hair, and regulates water passageways. It relates to the emotion of sadness and anxiety. It manifests itself in the nose.

Self-Testing Symptoms:

Dry cough	Chronic sore throat
Hoarse and low voice	Nose, throat, trachea discomfort
Dry mouth	Rhinitis, hay fever
Pimple, acne	Allergy, asthma, dermatitis, hives, cold
Facial speckles	Psoriasis
Skin disorder and rashes	
Constipation and dry stool	

Cleansing Formula (also known as Da Huang Qing Wei Wan)

According to traditional Chinese medicine, cleansing formula deals with stagnation of heat in the body due to blockage of chi and blood. Toxins accumulate in the body because of long-term imbalance of the meridians. Toxins also accumulate due to fatty, sugary, high-pressure blood and excessive food intake. This formula helps calm an overabundance of yang energy in the heart or lung meridians (yang disease) and stagnation of the spleen meridian (overacting of yang). It detoxifies the blood and digestive tracts.

Self-Testing Symptoms:

Swollen gums	Thirst, extreme dry mouth
Dry, cracked lips	Craving for cold drinks
Thick coating, dark red tongue	Constipation
Bad breath	Heartburn, stomach ache

You may wonder why specific symptoms are associated with the heart, liver, lung, kidney, and spleen meridian energy systems. For example, why do lungs relate to skin, kidney to bones and sexual essence, heart to spirit? In additional to traditional medicine, there is some scientific evidence. Research shows there are three layers of a human embryo. Common cells at embryo stage can be grown into different types of cells forming different parts of the body. A cell, such as one in the bone, is said to be of the same origin with another cell, say, from the kidney, if they are both originated from the cells in the same layer of an embryo. It turns out that kidney and bones are from the same origin. We also know that over millions of years of evolution, there has been a transition in living things from breathing primarily through the skin to breathing through the lungs. Thus, it is not difficult to realize that lung and skin are linked. We can also observe the connection, for example, between the heart and spirit; when in emotional stress, we stress our hearts, not our brains. Our heart pumps, aches, and hurts.

CHI-GONG BALANCING OF ENERGY

You can heal imbalance through herbs. But a more superior way is through chi-gong of mind and spirit. *The Yellow Emperor's Classic of Medicine* is the most authoritative book on traditional Chinese medicine, authored by the great Huang Di, the Yellow Emperor, who reigned 5,000 years ago. In it, there is the following dialog between Huang Di and his advisor Qi Bo:

Huang Di asked, "I have heard that in ancient times, when the sages treated, all they had to do was employ methods to guide and change the emotional and spiritual state of a person and redirect the energy flow. The sages utilized a method called zhu you, prayer, ceremony, and shamanism, which healed all conditions. Today, however, when doctors treat a patient, they use herbs to treat the internal aspect and acupuncture to treat the exterior. Yet some conditions do not respond. Why is this?"

Qi Bo answered, "In ancient times, people lived simply. They hunted, fished, and were with nature all day. When the weather cooled, they became active to fend off the cold. When the weather heated up in summer, they retreated to cool places. Internally, their emotions were calm and peaceful, and they were without excessive desires. Externally, they did not have the stress of today. They lived without greed and desire, close to nature. They maintained jing shen nei suo, or inner peace and concentration of the mind and spirit. This prevented the pathogens from invading. Therefore, they did not need herbs to treat their internal state, nor did they need acupuncture to treat the exterior. When they did contract disease they simply guided properly the emotions and spirit and redirected the energy flow, using the method of zhu you to heal the condition.

"People today are different. Internally, they are enslaved by their emotions and worries. They work too hard in heavy labor. They do not follow the rhythmic changes of the four seasons and thus become susceptible to the invasion of the thieves or winds. When their zheng, antipathogenic chi, is weak, pathogens invade to destroy the five zang organs, the bones, and the marrow. Externally, they are attacked via the sensory orifices, the skin, and muscles. Thus mild conditions become severe, and severe conditions turn fatal. At this point, the method of zhu you would be insufficient."[*]

As we discussed in Chapter 2, the human body forms its own microcosm, which is connected with the macrocosm of the universe. Chi in the human body travels through the meridians to support the life force in each cell of the body, and at the same time the chi exchanges with the external energies in the universe. When all meridians are open, chi can flow easily. Diseases cannot be accumulated. Energy is transported to all parts of the body. Energy is also absorbed through energy centers/acupuncture points from the outside. When the meridians are blocked, we get into trouble.

Chi-gong is a form of meditation. It is a way to train the body, mind, and spirit into a state of complete stillness. When at the extreme of stillness (extreme yin), movement (initial yang) oc-

---

[*] *The Yellow Emperor's Classic of Medicine*, translated by Maoshing Ni, Shambhala, 1995

curs. This movement is the chi in the body running through meridians as well as internal organs. Thus through chi-gong, we can open up all our meridian systems. We can also balance our systems.

Chi-gong is difficult. Not only are there many different chi-gong practices, but also combining spirit, mind, body, and channeling chi through meridians can be very challenging for some people. It penetrates every cell of us, goes far beyond the cellular biology level, works on the subtle energy body and the even higher spiritual energy body, and works with the cosmic energy of the universe beyond the human body. Therefore, chi-gong is a life-long learning journey. Nobody can claim they have attained the highest level of enlightenment. It is not the authors' intent to say they have. We believe that the more we accomplish in chi-gong, the more inadequate we feel.

It is very difficult to teach chi-gong in a book and it is important to have an enlightened teacher who can point out, based on each individual's specific situation, the right directions. Thus, in this section we only attempt to cover some basics that will help balance the meridians. For much deeper practice, we advise you to seek a truly enlightened master.

The first question: Is chi a real thing? Then we ask: Does chi really flow through the meridians and the organs as well as interact with the environment?

A pioneering researcher, the American physiologist Dr. Robert Wallace, conducted a series of experiments in the late 60's and 70's at UCLA that tell us something about chi. Meditators were studied over the span of a few years, and their biological and physiological data were recorded, such as brain waves, blood pressure, heart rate, etc.

It was discovered that meditators, after only a few minutes of meditation, entered into a state of deep relaxation, with slower heart beat due to decreased oxygen consumption. Metabolic rate was also dramatically reduced. Sleep can also achieve some of the same effects. However, sleep requires 4-6 hours instead of several minutes to reach the same state, and sleep only drops oxygen consumption by about 16% while it is twice as much in meditation.

Deep in the mountains of China, it is said Taoists spend many hours meditating without sleep and food. This is possible because meditation reaches a state much more rejuvenating than sleep, a state of increased chi. Due to the reduced metabolic rate, they need very little food, much like the hibernation state of bears in which the animal can sleep the whole winter without food, slowly burning the fat stored in the body for many months. Dr. Wallace called this "hypometabolic wakefulness."

Another study led by Dr. Wallace measured the meditators' biological age. Biological age is different from chronological age. People have the same chronological age, but could have a very different biological age. Biological age is the age at which your biological functions—blood pressure, hearing ability, eyesight, blood sugar, athletic ability—are compared to the average population of different ages. A 50-year-old may have a biological age of 30 because he or she functions like an average 30-year-old. Dr. Wallace's study showed that meditators as a group have a much younger biological age, by as much as 20 years.

The study also correlated years of meditation with aging improvement. Each year of meditation took off approximately one year of aging. Therefore, 20-year meditators, as a group average, can have as much as a 20-year younger biological age than their peer group, on the average. It was also shown that the effectiveness of meditation does not change relative to age. Hence, it is never too late to gain the effect. Of course, the right method of meditation is also very important.

A 1986 Blue Cross-Blue Shield Insurance study researched 2,000 meditators in Iowa. It was shown that the meditators as a group were much healthier than the average American population in 17 major diseases (they had 87% less   occurrence of severe heart disease and 50% less tumors).

One study conducted by Dr. Bernard Grad of McGill University in Canada produced interesting information about healers. Dr. Grad had started his research in "hands-on healing" during the 1960's. It was known that healers could lay their hands over diseased areas of patients without touching and create a healing effect. But it was not clear if it was due to the placebo effect (the power of the mind triggered by the patients' belief system).

Dr. Grad chose sick plants as the object of treatment to eliminate the impact of placebo, and a series of experiments were conducted. Healers were asked to hold bottles of water during their meditation to treat the water. Then sick plants were watered using plain water and treated water. Plants with treated water showed dramatically better growth and returned to health quickly. The study not only demonstrated the existence of a mysterious energy or chi (not directly measurable by modern technology), but also showed that water is a very good medium to store such energy. This shows why some healers can treat water and send the water hundreds of miles away to use in treating patients. It also shows the importance of drinking high-energy water, such as spring water, not only for its mineral content, but also for its energy content.

Scientific study of chi-gong has been extensively conducted in China, much earlier than in the U.S. There studies extend to the energy level and spiritual level. We will talk more about it in later chapters.

We'd like to take this opportunity to talk about science versus time-proven methods. There is significant benefit from chi-gong or meditation, both from the scientific point of view and from the ancient Chinese point of view. Many of us, raised in modern society, believe nothing but scientifically proven things. This is good and is the only way to weed out false claims. We believe in data and learned people. We believe in noted scientists and institutions, in science and technologies. However, there are some drawbacks to this belief system. For example, chi-gong has been around for 5,000 years in China. Our Chinese ancestors told us at that time that chi-gong is good for health, but it was not demonstrated in America scientifically until the 70's. The fundamental mechanism through which chi-gong works is still an unresolved scientific challenge. Should we wait until all is uncovered? We live for only a few decades as compared to what might take hundreds of years of scientific discovery.

If something is bogus, it would have been exposed through thousands of years and hundreds of generations of practicing and studying it. Therefore, something that survives that long must be close to the truth, the law of nature. Many aspects of this book are centered on the timelessness of thousands of years of wisdom rather than demanding fully understandable scientific proofs. In fact, many fashionable notions have been backed by "scientific data" and been found to be ineffective or have severe side effects.

The ancient Chinese referred to "blind people with the elephant." The story is that several blind men argued about what an elephant looked like. Each man was touching a different part of the elephant, some on the ear, some on the trunk, some on the tail. Nobody drew the right conclusion, but all were correct in their own perspectives. Nowadays, there is much scientific information behind every advertising campaign for new drugs and supplements. But it is difficult to understand the validity of the data. Therefore, we must balance our viewpoint between time-proven methods and scientifically proven methods.

THE ENERGY MERIDIANS

Chi (energy) flows through 12 principle and 8 extra meridians, and another 36 subordinate meridians. Each meridian passes through many acupuncture points, sometimes called energy centers. If chi stagnates through the meridians, blood sticks, spirit disperses, and essence is weakened. We must open all meridians to have vibrant health.

Du (yang) and Ren (yin) meridians are the most important. Du is a major meridian running on the back of the body. It is a yang energy meridian because it is facing to the sun when we have our hands on the ground. Ren is a major meridian on the front of the body. It belongs to the yin energy meridian. Du and Ren form a circle, called by the Chinese the microcosmic orbit. They connect through all major organ systems and main energy centers (acupuncture points).

In this section, we will talk about a simple method of opening and balancing the energy flows of Du and Ren meridians, or the microcosmic orbit, as well as the energy centers along the orbit.

Let's first talk about what exactly the Du and Ren meridians and the major energy centers are.

The Ren meridian has 24 acupuncture points along the front of the body. The next figure shows the major ones.

The following describes the location and function of a few major points. See the following diagram.

Ren1 (Huiyin)—Located midpoint between the anus and the penis or the vagina. This important energy point is called the "Gate of Life." It is the center point of yin energy in the body.

Ren4 (Guanyuan)—Located about midway between the naval and the pubic bone, about 1 and a half inches deep. This energy center is also called the "Ovarian Palace" (for woman) or the "Sperm Palace" (for man).

<u>Tan Tien</u>—Also referred to as lower Tan Tien, this is technically not a point on the Ren meridian, yet it is a most important chi-gong energy center. Located approximately 1 and a half inches inside the naval. *Tan* in Chinese means "pill" (of immortality); *Tien* means "field." Therefore, this is the energy field where the potent chi is collected. It is likened to the stove where gold is refined. The ancients believed that if our energy is highly refined through years of meditation, the chi will be strong enough for us to reach immortality.

Du and Ren Meridians

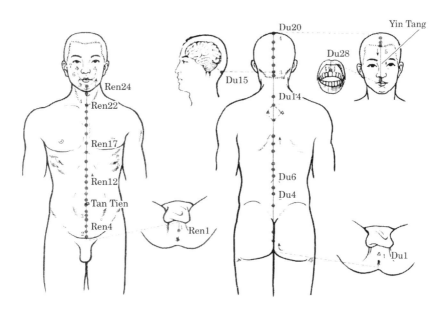

Ren12 (Zhongwan)—Located halfway between the sternum and the navel, also referred to as middle Tan Tien. This point is sometimes called the solar plexus. It controls spleen, adrenal, pancreas, and stomach.

Ren17 (Tanzhong)—Located between the nipples, a very important point, referred to as the heart center. The center relates to rejuvenation of love and joy. It controls the heart and lung.

Ren22 (Tiantu)—Located in the center of the suprasternal fossa (at the throat). This throat energy center relates to thyroid and parathyroid glands and regulates cough and asthma.

Ren24 (Chengjiang)—Located in the depression in the center of the mentolabial groove (between the lower lip and the chin). This is where the Ren meridian ends.

Now let's talk about Du meridian and the major energy centers. The Du meridian starts at Du1 (Changqiang) and runs through D4 (Mingmen), Du6 (Jizhong), Du14 (Dazhui), Du15 (Yamen), Du20 (Baihui), Yin Tang, and ends at Du28 (YinJiao).

Du1 (Changqiang)—Located midway between the tip of the coccyx and the anus. Called the passage to the door of life and death, this point is where the Ren meridian interacts with the Du meridian. Energy from Ren must transverse through this point to the Du meridian. If it is not open, energy is lost.

Du4 (Mingmen)—Located opposite the navel on the spine. *Ming* in Chinese means "life"; *men* means "gate." So this is the life gate, where kidney chi is concentrated. Kidney is where the prenatal chi is stored. The left kidney is yang, pertaining to the father; and the right kidney is yin, pertaining to the mother. Mingmen is the integration of yin and yang. It is one of the most important points in the body.

Du6 (Jizhong)—Located opposite the solar plexus (R12) on the spine. It relates to the adrenal gland, controlling the response of fight or flight, blood sugar, and sodium balance.

Du14 (Dazhui)—Located below the spinous process of the seventh cervical vertebra approximately at shoulder level (the big bone on the neck). It controls cough, asthma, neck pain, and back stiffness.

Du20 (Baihui)—Also called the crown, located above the mid-brain. Taoists believe that spirit enters us in the womb through the crown and it leaves from the crown when we die. The crown is open on newborns (soft on the head) and gradually closes as we age, closing the connection between humans and heaven. Advanced chi-gong requires reopening the crown.

Yin Tang—At the midpoint between the eyebrows, approximately 2 inches inside. This is a very important point, not officially a point on the Du meridian. It is referred to as the original cavity of the spirit, or the third eye, where the spirit sits in the advanced stage of chi-gong. It is a master center, regulating the pituitary and the pineal glands, controlling many life-force functions.

<u>Du28 (YinJiao)</u>—At the junction of the gum and the frenulum of the upper lip. This is the end of Du meridian.

Microcosmic orbit starts at Tan Tien and ends at Tan Tien. It follows the path of Tan Tien, Ren4, Ren1, Du1, Du4, Du6, Du14, Du20, Yin Tang, Ren22, Ren17, Ren12, Tan Tien. Note that the natural flow of yin meridians (such as Ren) goes downward and the flow of yang meridians (such as Du) goes upward.

OPENING AND BALANCING MERIDIANS

In this section, we will talk about opening and balancing the microcosmic orbit. Please note that here we present chi-gong which uses the mind to concentrate each point in order to connect body, mind, and spirit to strike open the energy centers. The purpose is to provide a method that millions of people can practice to achieve better health. However, this is not the ideal way to teach advanced chi-gong. The advanced Taoist chi-gong requires us to first achieve complete stillness—no form, no substance, no body, and no thought. According to the principle of change, when stillness is achieved (when yin is at its extreme), yang is born and movement occurs. This movement is the original stirring of the chi, which automatically blows open the energy meridians. Since this is very difficult without face-to-face teaching from an enlightened teacher, it is not practical to cover it here.

We present instead an elementary routine which will nevertheless dramatically improve health.

<u>Basic Positions</u>: Start in a sitting position, with Du20 (crown) and Ren1 (Huiyin) vertically aligned, feet flat on the ground. Rest both hands on the lap, with left hand under right hand, left thumb in the right palm, and right thumb

pressing on the back of left hand between thumb and index finger. Slightly close the eyes. Touch the upper palate with the tongue to connect the Du and Ren meridians. This is similar to connecting two electrical circuits. Breathe in and out very slowly, continuously, and lightly, as though there were no breath—1 to 4 ins and outs per minute. Don't count it or force yourself. It's all natural. Inhale into the lower belly, fill it up toward the lung. The mind is completely empty. Keep this throughout the whole exercise.

Opening Energy Centers: When still and empty, move concentration to the Tan Tien. Practice for several days until you can feel sensation (such as warm, numbness, tingling, vibration). When Tan Tien is open, continue to open other points. Move concentration to R4, Ren1, Du1, Du4, Du6, Du14, Du20, Yin Tang, Ren22, Ren17, Ren12, Tan Tien. At each point, stay for a few minutes until you feel the chi.

Always finish each session at Tan Tien by concentrating at Tan Tien for a little longer (5-10 minutes), accumulating chi and storing it in Tan Tien. It is risky to let chi stagnate at other points, especially points on the chest and the head. Care must be taken to return the energy to Tan Tien.

Circling the Microcosmic Orbit: Once all energy centers on the microcosmic orbit (Du and Ren meridians) are open, you can use one breath to draw the energy all the way from Hui Yin through the Du meridian up to the crown, and then breathe out to send the chi down through Ren meridian back to Tan Tien. Thus each breath in and out completes a whole circle of the microcosmic orbit.

Yang Emerges from Extreme Yin: As your practice becomes more mature and your microcosmic orbit is completely open, you do not have to concentrate through each point. Just achieve an extreme still and empty state. Chi will automatically flow. However, make sure always to end the session of chi-gong back at Tan Tien.

Practice every day for at least thirty minutes. As you become more experienced, you can reach a chi-gong state at any time, in meetings, waiting in line, sitting at a dinner table, watching TV. Chi-gong becomes part of you and your life, not just limited to practice time. Continued sessions keep your main meridians balanced and open, accumulate chi, and make you stronger and healthier.

With open meridians and energy centers, you will feel extremely comfortable when performing chi-gong—a feeling of intoxication that you don't want to end. You will feel every cell of your body breathing, opening and closing. You will feel as if your physical form is disappearing. You will immerse with the vast universe. You will co-exist with the infinite energy source of the universe. Your microcosm will merge with the macrocosm of heaven and earth.

APPLYING THE PROTOCOL

We all have imbalance in our energy systems because we are constantly pushed out of equilibrium due to daily problems of living. The effect of imbalance accumulates. Longer-term imbalance will shut off energy centers and block meridians. Chinese medicine believes that many diseases are a result of the accumulation of imbalance. Imbalances build little by little without any notice until becoming uncontrollable, such as with cancer. This protocol helps make sure that we always come back to the optimal balance of energy systems. This balancing has to be done often so we can make many small corrections instead of very large ones.

To begin, perform the symptom test of the Eight Fundamental Formulas. Choose the formulas corresponding to your symptoms. You can start by concentrating on the formula where you have a severe symptom. You can also take a formula where you have 2-3 less severe symptoms. Use the herbs to rebalance the system for 100 days to rejuvenate all the cells of the body back to balance. These herbal formulas have been known for hundreds of years and are available from most Chinese herbal medicine stores as well as our PingClinic (www.pingclinic.com).

Use microcosmic orbit chi-gong to open and balance energy meridians. Try to perform this every day for at least thirty minutes. Make it part of your daily life so you can accumulate time in the chi-gong state.

Having finished working on the energy plane, we now move on to the spiritual plane.

CHAPTER 7

FIFTH PROTOCOL: PRESERVE SPIRIT ENERGY

My best friend, Justin, called. He was in town and wanted to have dinner with me. It would be good to see my old college friend, who came from one of the most remote and poorest villages in China, probably the first to enter college in the long history of the village. He is smart, intuitive, naïve, truthful, real. There is no pretending in his manner. The first time he showed up in the dorm, after a 50-mile walk carrying his luggage to save bus fare, he was barefoot, shirtless, sweaty, with dirt covering his boyish face. He graduated first in our class, receiving a Ph.D. in physics from Stanford, yet never displayed any arrogance, jealousy, anger, aggressiveness, or greediness, qualities typically associated with modern men. It still impresses me today. For a big city girl like me and most of our classmates, he was different, natural and unspoiled.

"What are you doing these days, Justin?" I asked after picking our menu items in the Chinese restaurant.

"After graduation I read about An Wang, you know, the founder of Wang Laboratories. He inspired me to get into big business. So I joined General Electric. Now I am a vice president, running this $900 million electronics business. I have about 3500 people working in my division." Justin still talked in his villager's manner.

"I am impressed," I said, "but cannot imagine how you managed to climb a corporate ladder. I have heard that there is a lot of politics to deal with, just like in the Congress in Washington, D.C."

"Well, yes. When you get to this level, people naturally are very competitive. They fight for power, compete to get credit for success, socialize to build alliances, and cling together in little cliques to get ahead. You don't have to be wrong to be wrong. Remember the stories about the kingdoms in the Warring Period of China. That was when the greatest strategists such as Sun Tzu were created."

"But I cannot put a village boy and a large corporate executive together," I said. "How did you learn all of this? You must have given up all your original nature in order to be successful in such a modern corporation."

"Yes, I had to learn all of this, which at times, is very stressful. I must fit into the corporate image—a different person from myself—strong, elegant, eloquent, knowledgeable all the time regardless of the truth. My mind has to think a million things all at once every minute, every day, even in my sleep. I so much long for life in my home village, where I could catch fishes, collect bamboo shoots, hunt wild chickens, climb on the trees to get berries. In those days, I spent a lot of time staring at the sky and dreaming, as though my whole body and mind dissolved into the stars. I craved nothing because I had everything in the village."

"How do you handle this?"

"I figured out a way. I decided to live two lives simultaneously. Each day at work, I am the corporate executive, most competitive in everything I do. Off work, I am the poor village boy again. My mind is calm and empty. My body is relaxed. I don't watch movies and TV because it raises my emotions. All that divorce, violence, sex, suspense, power, fame, and wealth taints my mind. Being able to switch back and forth at ease makes me very happy. My life is great. I have the benefit of both worlds. I sometimes feel that I am the magic monkey in the old Chinese novels who could change at will to any form, any face, any mind. It makes me very spiritual."

"Amazing," I exclaimed. "I am sure many people want to do this."

Ping's Diary

Aging is due to two major fundamental causes: the leakage of vital essence (such as semen, blood, enzymes, hormones, body fluids) and the leakage of spirit energy through emotions and stress. When both essence and spirit energy are reduced, the life-sustaining chi is weakened. However, before puberty, neither leak is substantial. Therefore, the body builds itself toward becoming a higher energy being. Between birth and age 16, the human system is in negative entropy. Recall our discussion in Chapter 2 on the laws of living and the laws of thermodynamics: entropy is the state of disorganization. Negative entropy indicates a system moving toward more and more organization. A more-organized system has more long-lasting potential. After puberty, we are in positive entropy as we move toward aging and a deteriorating energy potential due to the two deadly leaks of essence and spirit.

This chapter will discuss how to stop the spiritual energy leakage and is the first chapter to deal with our spiritual energy plane. Remember, spiritual healing is superior and immortal, energy healing is the next, food healing is excellent and promotes long living, natural herb healing is good, and chemical/surgery healing is the last resort.

THE TREND TOWARD SPIRIT ENERGY LEAKAGE

We live in a world that grows busier and busier. We evolved from the very slow pace of life in small villages or tribes to modern cosmopolitan life. People in remote tribes are not bombarded with news. They have simple social standards, simple jobs, mostly related to the basic activities of making a living (hunting, farming, etc.), and a simple life. Money is not that useful. Even if they had money, there is nowhere to spend it. Fame is confined to a very small circle. Lust is not within the social/tribal standard. Power is more absolute from the tribal leaders. There are simply not enough things for people to crave and fight for. Time flows slowly. After dark, there is no electricity. People sit around chatting and watching stars. The mind works slowly because speed is not needed. As long as people can make a basic living, there is nothing else available to seek.

In contrast, in modern life there is so much to be desired. We want more money, a bigger house, better cars, vacations, travel, better jobs, career advancement, power, and fame and to indulge in sex, food, and play. The efficient information flow due to modern technology (newspaper, transportation, Internet, database, TV, radio) has overpowered us with all kinds of opportunities to seek and crave more. Every minute we are presented with opportunities which lure us to work harder. We hear news of an economic slowdown and crank up our computers to sell stocks. We see ads on the Internet for jobs which give us hope for better-paying positions and suddenly find ourselves in the job-interviewing process. We hear about sales at a supermarket and hurry out to buy. We become angry when co-workers take credit for something we've done and boast to our bosses. We are sued because others simply want to make some extra dollars. We get ticketed for speeding, angry with our car dealers, and anxious when the lawn and trees are drying up because the sprinkler is broken.

But even this is not enough excitement, so we watch movies that are suspenseful, violent, sexual, and highly emotional. All of this stimulates emotional stress. There is just too much; every minute of our lives is occupied. How many times are our brain cells buzzing, compared with people in primitive tribes? We'd bet over a million times. It would be a nice research project to find out.

Here are some statistics on modern stress.

- It is reported that more than 10% of the population has been diagnosed with some form of mental illness (schizophrenia, phobias, depression, or anxiety disorders).
- *The Journal of the American Medical Association, JAMA,* reported in 1998 that up to 24% of adults experience a mental-health crisis in any given year.
- In 1995, 5-6 million Americans suffered from obsessive compulsive disorder, yet fewer than 20% sought help (*Cosmopolitan, MDX Health Digest,* 1995).
- NARSAD Research Newsletter reported in 1996 that 7-14% of children will experience an episode of major depression before age 15.
- *Drug Topics* reported in 1996 that the most popular form of antidepressants, serotonin reuptake inhibitors (SSRIs), account for over 40,133,000 prescriptions each year, costing consumers over $3 billion annually, a gain of some 35% per year.
- It was stated in a 1992 Department of Health and Human Services report that psychiatric hospitals increased inpa-

tient admissions from 46.2 per 100,000 population in 1969 to over 156 per 100,000 population in 1988, and during the same period of time outpatient additions increased from 12.8 per 100,000 to 51.2 per 100,000.

- Suicide was the fifth leading cause of years of potential life lost before the age of 65, reported *JAMA*, August, 1995.

No doubt we are living in a world that is exciting but usually stressful, especially if we don't know how to handle it. It is impossible for most of us to have the luxury of not working or only partially working or to have a slower pace of life to preserve our health.

As mentioned earlier, one interesting set of data is how life insurance companies evaluate people's premiums. Insurance companies have to do a good job of estimating the risk of death because that is how they make money. One aspect of the premium estimate is to classify people into categories of what they do for a living. It's interesting that the following are listed as life-extending occupations: symphony orchestra conductor, scientist and mathematician, university professor, successful creative artist, U.S. government employee. As you can see, these occupations happen to be ones with less stress as compared with corporate executives, athletes, dot.com company employees, small business owners, or politicians. Those with less stress can immerse themselves in their specialties (such as math), their enjoyment (orchestra conductor), and their unconscious mind creativity (artists), highly concentrating their minds on a single subject in which they can by and large forget about things happening around them. These are usually jobs not involving stressful deadlines or complex political maneuvers or power struggles.

Growing emotional distress is a phenomenon spanning thousands of years of human evolution. It is not a new problem, except that today it is more intensified. An interesting dialog can be found in *The Yellow Emperor's Classic of Medicine*. The following dialog took place between the Huang Di and his advisor Qi Bo:

> Huang Di asked, "I've heard that in the days of old everyone lived one hundred years without showing the usual signs of aging. In our time, however, people age prematurely, living only fifty years. Is this due to a change in the environment, or is it because people have lost the correct way of life?"
>
> Qi Bo replied, "In the past, people practiced the Tao, the Way of Life. They understood the principle of balance, of yin and yang, as presented by the transformation of the energies of the universe. Thus, they formulated practices such as Dao-in, an exercise combining stretching, massaging, and breathing to promote energy flow, and meditation to help maintain and harmonize themselves with the universe. They ate a balanced diet at regular times, arose and retired at regular hours, avoided overstressing their bodies and minds, and refrained from overindulgence of all kinds. They maintained well being of body and mind; thus, it is not surprising that they lived over one hundred years.
>
> "These days, people have changed their way of life. They drink wine as though it were water, indulge excessively in destructive activities, drain their jing—the body's essence that is stored in the kidneys—and deplete their chi. They do not know the secret of conserving their energy and vitality. Seeking emotional excitement and momentary pleasures, people disregard the natural rhythm and order of the universe. They fail to regulate their lifestyle and diet, and sleep improperly. So it is not surprising that they look old at fifty and die soon after.

"The accomplished ones of ancient times advised people to guard themselves against gu zei feng, disease-causing factors. On the mental level, one should remain calm and avoid excessive desires and fantasies, recognizing and maintaining the natural purity and clarity of the mind. When internal energies are able to circulate smoothly and freely, and the energy of the mind is not scattered but is focused and concentrated, illness and disease can be avoided.

"Previously, people led a calm and honest existence, detached from undue desire and ambition; they lived with an untainted conscience and without fear. They were active, but never depleted themselves. Because they lived simply, these individuals knew contentment, as reflected in their diet of basic but nourishing goods and attire that was appropriate to the season but never luxurious. Since they were happy with their position in life, they did not feel jealousy or greed. They had compassion for others and were helpful and honest, free from destructive habits. They remained unshakable and unswayed by temptations, and they were able to stay centered even when adversity arose. They treated others justly, regardless of their level of intelligence or social position."[*]

THE TAOIST VIEW OF EMOTION

In the classic *Cultivating Stillness*, written in the era between 220-589 C.E. by Lao Tzu, who was the father of Taoism, we find the following teaching about human nature, spirit, and mind:

If people can constantly be pure and still, then heaven and earth will return to their places. The spirit tends toward purity, but the mind disturbs it. The mind tends toward stillness but it

---

[*] *The Yellow Emperor's Classic of Medicine,* translated by Maoshing Ni, Shambhala, 1995.

is opposed by craving. If you are able to control desire, then the mind will be still. Clear the mind and the spirit will be pure. Those who are unable to attain the Tao are those whose minds are not clear and who are still slaves of their emotions. Look into your mind and there is no mind. Look at appearances and appearances have no forms. Gaze at distant objects and objects do not exist. Understand these three modes of cognition and you will see emptiness.[*]

In the first sentence of this quote, heaven refers to spirit and earth refers to essence in the microcosm of the human body. In its prenatal state, the two are united. Yin and yang are together. Mind and body are one. This oneness represents the original higher vibrating energy. It stays young and lasts long. In the postnatal state, yin and yang become separated. Life becomes limited. Life now follows the law of life discussed in Chapter 2. Therefore, Lao Tzu said that if we can really achieve a state of mind of stillness and emptiness, we can unit the spirit, chi, and essence and become immortal. People cannot achieve this due to craving, desire, and emotions.

In traditional Chinese medicine, there are seven deadly emotions. These are the emotions of overjoy, anger (rage), sadness, pensiveness (overly thoughtful), grief, fear, and fright. Each of these emotions is considered harmful to the body's energy systems. They weaken spirit energy. The ancient Chinese believed that the natural leakage of spiritual energy flows upward. Each flush of emotion reduces our spiritual energy reserve. Through a lifelong process of overjoy, anger, sadness, pensiveness, grief, fear, and fright, we gradually deplete ourselves of our spiritual energy reserve. Thus we grow older and older following the path of

---

[*] *Cultivating Stillness*, Lao Tzu, translated by Eva Wong, Shambhala, Boston & London, 1992.

the law of life. Emotions are also related to the five major organ meridian systems. They block and weaken these systems.

Body, mind, and spirit are all connected. For example, heart is the master of spirit—this is very different from Western medicine where heart is considered merely a blood pump. When a musician's heart is transplanted to a person, the person is found to have more inclination to music. When the mind is frustrated, the heart feels uncomfortable. When a person is kind and loving, we often say this person has a good heart. So it is extremely important to realize that emotions, mind, and the different parts of the body are connected.

Overjoy is related to heart energy. The expression "dying laughing" means people die during intense laughter because they strike the heart too hard. When overjoyed, the heart needs to pump blood hard to fuel the joy. It scatters the heart energy or chi. Joy at its normal level is healthy. If we have an optimistic outlook of life and are naturally happy and joyful, it warms the heart and cheers the spirit. However, taken to the extreme, it is very harmful and needs to be avoided. Fright is the opposite of overjoy. Fright is due to a sudden change of environment. It strikes the heart. It disturbs the spirit.

Anger is very bad for liver energy. It causes stagnation of chi and of blood. We often see people's faces turn blue or white and eyes turn red when they are in extreme rage. We see people shake with rage. Liver is the organ system which manufactures and stores blood. When liver chi is impaired due to anger, blood and chi circulation is interrupted. One of our patients had periodic headaches. Every few weeks, he would get a sinus infection, sore throat, gum pain, sore eyes, and headaches. Upon diagnosis, it was discovered that he frequently went through very stressful situations. His temper built up over time.

When the anger accumulates, it turns into liver yang imbalance, as discussed in the preceding chapter. The extra yang due to anger flares up to cause all the symptoms. In Western medicine, it would be called inflammation. At each outburst of this imbalance, the body fights hard and returns back to balance until the accumulation becomes too large again.

Sadness hurts the lung energy. When people are extremely sad, they weep and have difficulty catching their breath. When lung energy is blocked, people usually feel oppressed in the chest and depressed. Excessive grief also impacts the digestion process and injures the lungs. It leads to the dejection or stagnation of lung chi, leading to hypofunctioning of internal organs. That is why we see people with excessive grief having difficulty breathing, suffocation in the chest, listlessness, and depression.

Excessive pensiveness injures the spleen. It is said in the ancient Chinese classic *Plain Questions*, "The spleen is the organ that stores intention and shares control of determination; with the heart, it decides everything." The spleen system is also responsible for transporting nutrients and water throughout the body. Thus prolonged excessive pensiveness impairs the digestive system. One simple experiment is to do some very hard thinking while eating dinner. You can feel the impact on digestion. Unfortunately, dining has become one of the important means of conducting business or other high-pressure social events which require hard thinking—taking the mind away from enjoying food.

Fear affects kidney energy, due to hypofunctioning of internal organ systems. It causes nightmares and bad dreams.

The root causes of the seven deadly emotions of overjoy, anger, sadness, pensiveness, grief, fear, and fright are usually caused by the desire and cravings for power, wealth, fame, food, and sex. These desires have been intensified in our materialistic world. For example, there are many opportunities to make money and unlimited places to spend money. There is always something to buy. There are more and more things to crave as materialism advances. The Internet, TV, magazines, books, and radio lead our emotions in all sorts of directions.

Emotions due to worldly craving are one of the major root causes of poor health and accelerated aging. We'll talk in later sections about how to reduce such spiritual energy leakage in order to preserve youthfulness.

MODERN SCIENCE'S VIEW OF EMOTION

Modern science looks at emotion, craving, and desire from the point of view of stress. There is no doubt that severe emotion creates stress, and craving and desire for things creates emotion.

There is a strong link between emotion and hormones. The master gland of hormones is the pituitary, sitting behind the eyes inside the brain. It controls the release of many hormones, including the growth hormones. When emotions arise, hormones are affected and a series of physiological responses occur. When you are fed up with a person who is seeking a loving relationship, you immediately are "turned off" (of all your sexual hormones). Many women, for example, find that being anxious or upset may delay menstruation.

It works the other way also. When hormones change, emotions rise. The hormones estrogen and progesterone, which control menstrual cycles, may have a profound influence on a woman's mood. Therefore, emotions and hormones are paired. When emotions rise, the normal body physiological process is altered. Since it is not natural, meaning it is influenced by outside factors (or craving for outside factors), the influence is usually against the normal body balance and pulls the body away from its equilibrium.

There are two major hormones involved in stressful situations. The first, adrenaline, is secreted by adrenal glands sitting on top of the kidneys. This is the so-called fright and flight hormone.

The release of adrenaline is nature's way to deal with physical threat and psychological stress. It is tightly connected to the nervous system. When a dangerous or stressful situation arises, there is a surge in the production of adrenaline, which makes the heart beat faster and harder to pump blood. Simultaneously, it restricts blood vessels near the surface of the body and the gut so that more blood can be supplied to the heart. Thus, it shuts down the stomach or the digestion process, and turns our face white. As a result, blood pressure is greatly raised. Adrenaline also raises the blood sugar level by accelerating the conversion of glycogen stored in the liver and the muscles. This is to prepare the extra energy required in a fight and flight situation. It also stimulates the lungs to breathe harder to supply more oxygen for higher fuel burning, dilates the pupils, dries the mouth, and causes sweating.

Now let's think about prolonged stress. Many of us spend long workdays in stressful environments competing in the market economy, doing good work, earning promotions, making more money, and achieving recognition. We then spend our dinner time socializing to build relationships with people important to our work or to get a deal done with business partners. Before we go to bed, we take care of our children and family chores. The next day, we are in the same cycle again. Modern life has turned our stress hormone from an occasional hormone to a constant one.

Why does it matter? Because the stress hormone causes abnormal responses in the body: high blood pressure, high blood sugar, restricted circulation of blood to the surface of the body, and the shutdown of the digestive process and other body functions. The digestive system does not function properly and nutrition is not well absorbed. Blood sugar is high and insulin rises, making us fat and more prone to diabetes. Just note the statistics: from 1990 to 1998, diabetes jumped 33%, 70% in the 30-39 age group, 40% in 40-49 age group, and 31% in 50-59 age group, according to data provided by the Centers for Disease Control and Prevention. By age 50, one in ten Americans have diabetes and many more have a blood sugar level at the high end of the "normal" range defined by the medical professions. Also according to the latest national statistics, 61% of American adults are overweight as defined by a body mass index over 25 (BMI = metric weight divided by the square of metric height).

The second stress-related hormone is cortisone, also produced by the adrenal glands.   It is sometimes called the sugar hormone because it is responsible for raising the blood sugar level. There are several hormones which elevate blood sugar level, but there is only one which reduces sugar level: insulin. When the sugar level is constantly raised, insulin becomes deficient or the ability for insulin to bind to cells becomes deficient. In such cases, diabetes results. Under stress, cortisone stimulates the conversion of protein to blood sugar in order to increase the fuel to fight the stressful situation. That protein is mostly derived from the breakdown of muscle tissue; thus, chronically elevated cortisone leads to accelerated muscle reduction. Furthermore, it is also a major cause of bone mass loss. It is basically a catabolic (the process of breaking down things in the body) hormone that tears down tissue and bones in order to raise the blood sugar level.

Medically we use cortisone for many emergency situations. Asthmatic children can easily catch a cold and develop severe breathing problems. Many times use of cortisone or a cortisone-like medicine will immediately relieve the emergency situation. This is because cortisone works to reduce inflammation. However, a constant release of cortisone from the body due to stressful situations or the intake of externally administered cortisone is actually immuno-suppressive and toxic to the thymus—the master organ responsible for immune functions. In addition, chronic high levels of cortisone interfere with the building of muscles and cartilage, damage neurons leading to memory loss, and can cause poor brain function. Some theories of female adult acne also place the blame on cortisone for the aging effects of skin due to a period of prolonged stress.

For the body to produce cortisone, it uses the main precursor hormone pregnenolone to make glucocorticoids. But the same precursor hormone is also used to make DHEA, the antioxidant hormone, as well as other important anti-aging hormones such as progesterone and testosterone. Thus, constant stress resulting in constant production of cortisone reduces the production of other very useful hormones. Elevated cortisone also means lower production of the thyroid hormones, so important for the regulation of metabolism. This further accelerates the aging process.

DHEA, widely touted as a hormone to combat oxidants and keep the body healthy and young, is our built-in defense against excess cortisone. In fact, most of the benefit of DHEA can be explained in terms of its role as an inhibitor of the biological actions of corticosteroids. Some anti-aging doctors believe that the ratio between cortisone and DHEA is a good measure of aging. Under stress, the production of cortisone is higher, whereas the production of DHEA is lower. Thus, chronic stress raises the ratio and accelerates aging.

Interestingly, in men there is a clear antagonistic relationship between insulin and DHEA. Lowering insulin (whether through carbohydrate-restricted diet or through insulin-lowering drugs such as Metformin) creates dramatically higher DHEA levels. In both sexes, meditation not only lowers cortisone, but also raises DHEA.

In summary, adrenalin and cortisone are basically "emergency hormones." They are meant to help us survive a life-or-death emergency and then to be quickly cleared out of the body. Chronic elevated levels of adrenaline and cortisone caused by the constant stress of daily life inhibit the normal functioning of the body and accelerate aging.

PRESERVING SPIRIT ENERGY

You may now be wondering, is it possible to avoid all the harmful emotions? How can we reduce daily stress? How can we keep adrenaline and cortisone levels reasonably low?

Obviously it's impossible to eliminate all stress, nor would it be necessarily desirable if we want to continue living in this modern world. It is not desirable to hide in the mountains like the ancient sages. We don't always have the luxury of choosing where we want to work. We have to push ourselves hard, or be pushed to work hard. We have to feed our families; drive through smog-filled congested freeways; deal with politics, laws, and social standards, all somewhat unnaturally forced upon us. We feel the need to buy brand-name clothing for our kids and strive for better cars, houses, education, restaurants, social status, power, money, and fame.

This is how most of us function in busy modern everyday life. We are busier than the bees, stressed to the extreme, and keep building up the pressure.

But, yes, there is a way to have emotion without depleting our spiritual energy and depriving ourselves of our young vibrant life!

To understand how we can rid ourselves of stress, we must understand the cumulative effect of the body, mind, and spirit. Emotional stress is a positive feedback system, which is an unstable system. In the automatic control theory, a negative control is a stable system. In a negative control system, a reference signal is provided (such as the desired room temperature in the air conditioning control panel). When the output (the actual room temperature) is higher than the desired setting, AC is turned on to lower the temperature. Here the negative control is that the control action is in the opposite direction (lower the temperature) of the actual (higher temperature). On the other hand, a positive control system is unstable. Its control action is in the same direction of the output. An example of this would be a control that keeps the AC off and the heater on as the room temperature becomes higher and higher than the desired level, until it is too hot in the room. Similarly, stress is also a positive feedback system. The longer we are in a stressful mood, the more deteriorated our overall spiritual health.

Here is an everyday example. We see a co-worker in a bad mood. He must have had a bad experience, such as being skipped over for a promotion. Because of it, he looks at everything from a dark side. It now appears to him that everything is against him. This ever-spiraling elevation of emotional stress can be explained easily through the viewpoint of traditional Chinese medicine.

Anger affects your eating and sleeping. It drains energy. It impairs your liver energy system, since anger is the emotion that impairs the liver the most. When the liver is impaired, you become irritable because the liver relates to the emotion of anger and depression. According to the five-element theory, liver is wood. It promotes fire (heart). If liver is weak, heart energy is also impaired. Liver produces blood, and the heart transports blood. When the heart is weak, you become restless and sleepless. Your spirit becomes a wanderer. But heart is fire and it promotes earth (spleen). Therefore heart weakness affects the health of the spleen system. Nutrients cannot be converted and absorbed effectively. You tire easily, both physically and mentally. This makes you more depressed. Spleen is earth and it promotes metal (lung). With the lung system impaired, you fall victim to allergy, flu, cold, cough, asthma. Your anxiety is high. Since lung is metal, it promotes water (kidney), so your kidney energy is weakened. You become more hesitant. Your bones and joints are weak, and your marrows are lacking. You become impotent and lose hair. As kidney is water, it promotes wood (liver).

You have made one big circle: from chronic anger to liver, to heart, to spleen, to lung, to kidney, back to liver—a destructive circle through all five major organ energy systems.   Long-term stress builds up until it destroys your health and depletes your spirit energy.   *Therefore, we must learn how to release stress instantaneously.   Never let it accumulate.*   It is far too dangerous to health and longevity.

A MEDITATION TO ELIMINATE STRESS

When our body is dirty, we bathe.   When our teeth are dirty, we brush them.   When we eat dirty food, we need detoxification to cleanse our blood and digestive tract.   When we get fat, we hurry to lose weight.   When our body contracts a bacterial infection, we use antibiotics to flush it out.

All these are nothing compared to the dirtiness of emotional stress, the root cause of declining health.   We need a spiritual and mental cleanup to improve health and longevity.

We should be able to sleep well, free of night dreams.   We must not let stress accumulate even one day.   A very effective solution is pre-bedtime meditation.   This resets the mind and spirit, detoxifies all the emotional stress of the day, calms the mind for a good night's sleep, and renews you for the next day.   The following is a simple routine.   Perform it nightly for 30 minutes before sleep.

Pre-bedtime Meditation: Start in a sitting position, with Du20 (crown at the top of the head) and Ren1 (Huiyin –midpoint between the anus and the penis or the vagina) vertically aligned.   Place feet flat on the ground.   Rest both hands on the lap, with left hand under right hand, left thumb in the right palm, and right thumb pressing on the back of left hand between thumb and index finger. Close your eyes. Touch the upper palate with the tongue to connect the Du and Ren meridians, similar to connecting two electrical circuits. Breathe in and out very slowly about 1-4 times per minute. Start in the lower belly, filling up toward the lungs. Relax the whole body, every muscle, tendon, ligament, bone. Look internally at Tan Tien (inside the navel). Listen to the breath going in and out. Completely empty the mind—absolutely no thoughts, no form, no imagination. Everything is super-natural through complete immersion into the vast universe.

This turns weak into strong, dispersed into concentrated, degenerated into vibrant, impotent into vitality. It reunites the three treasures, the spirit, chi, and essence. You must achieve ab-solute stillness of body (relax) and mind (empty).

Your hands will be warm. Your body will be in a harmo-nious state—chi and blood bring warmth throughout every part of the body. Your mind and spirit will feel so luxuriously comfort-able, almost intoxicated, that you won't ever want to leave this state of relaxation.

Almost all stress and emotions are a result of some sort of craving and desire, for money, power, fame, material goods (house, cars), sex and love, food, etc. Most of the time, you work so hard for things that even if you ultimately get them, you do not really have the time to enjoy them. How often have we heard about a father who worked hard his entire life, retired at 60, believ-ing his dreams had come true, and then died suddenly from a heart attack. Such a pity. A lifetime of accumulation with enjoyment cut short. We often see old people suffering with degenerative dis-eases. What is the use of fame, power, money, sex, and food if our health cannot be maintained? Many times we see the rich and fa-mous become old and lose living ability (Alzheimer's disease, stroke). Sometimes nobody cares about them anymore, not even family members.

We arrive in the world naked. We leave the world naked too. We bring nothing to the world, and we can take nothing away. The things in our worldly life are both real and perceived. The real achievement of life is determined a priori by your fate. In Einstein's relativity theory, space and time are relative. Future events can be seen in the present. Thus, in the relative sense, the future events have already been determined. We should try our best to do good work, participating in our desired career. If it is meant to be ours, it will be ours. If it is not ours, it is not going to be ours. If we are rich, it's great. It's meant to be that way. If we are famous, great. But if we are not, so be it. It is our destiny.

There is an old Chinese saying that "planning of success is humanly possible, but true success depends on the heavenly power." At the end of Han Dynasty (around 200 A.D.), China was divided into three kingdoms, Chu, Wu, and Wuei. There was a deciding battle, which could have helped Chu to unify the whole country. The commander of Chu lured the Wuei troops onto a road through a deep canyon with huge cliffs on both sides. The Chu army then blocked the escape routes and set fire to the whole canyon, shooting arrows and stones at the Wuei troops. It seemed the Wuei troops had no chance for survival. The commander of Wuei, a very talented warrior, sighed about "heaven's desire to terminate me." Suddenly, out of the blue sky, a gusty wind brought a huge rainstorm, which completely extinguished the fire. The Wuei troops fought their way out of the canyon and escaped. Later, Wuei became stronger and unified the whole country into the Jin Dynasty.

The moral of the story is that although the Chu commander tried his best and did a superior job in strategy, he still could not unite the country. Thus, "planning for success is humanly possible, but true success depends on the heavenly power." We may dream of becoming a millionaire overnight, we may want a promotion badly, we may desire the fame of movie stars. But all we need to do is to try our best. If it comes, it is really meant to belong to us. If it does not come, it is not meant to be. Emotion and worry do not help anything if everything is pre-arranged. Many times, emotion does not solve anything but makes you miserable, not just temporarily feeling terrible but permanently marring your health.

The perception of life is very important. When we reach a state of mind and spirit where we can look at things in the plainest way, we have attained a much higher plateau of spiritual development. We will be rid of a large toxic factor to health—the emotional stress.

All of us have our own original nature, very comfortable in one way or another. However, we have to be a little out of our nature in order to be successful in the modern business or social world. Some of us are innately quiet, but we have to stretch our neck out there to speak publicly. Some of us like loose casual clothing because it is comfortable, but we have to dress for success by strangling ourselves with neckties and squeezing our feet into hard leather shoes. Some of us don't like a few of our co-workers, but we have to say good things about them and be charming at social dinners.

Some of us don't enjoy working too hard but still do it because we have to. Some of us don't like having to leash our dogs on the beach, but we have to follow the rule. Some of us like natural milk straight from the cow, orange juice right out of the squeeze. But we cannot find them in the supermarket. They may even be unlawful. It is the modern world. We are part of it. On one hand, it is great to live in such a world, but on the other we have to denature ourselves a lot. But denaturing ourselves all the time is deadly to our health and longevity. If we can develop an ability to switch between two lives, natured and denatured, then we can separate into two segments, two co-existing lives.

Imagine that you are two completely different persons every day. On one hand, during working hours you are competitive, hardworking, social, driving—a success in every way. On the other hand, during off hours and weekends, you are a natural person—casual, honest, naïve, yourself, simple, relaxed, slow-paced, easygoing, free spirited, calm-minded, quiet, unrestricted—the epitome of primitive original nature. You don't answer cell phones, get onto work computer networks, socialize for the sake of work, do business travel, or worry about work. In essence, you have completely separated the two lives. You now can live two lives independently—one in the competitive worldly materialistic realm, the other in the still, emotionless, stressless, empty-minded spiritual realm. This is the only way to preserve our spirit, the highest energy source of life. If you can indeed achieve such a state of mind and lifestyle, you can easily reset your stress to zero every day. You will find so much more enjoyment of what original life is supposed to offer.

APPLYING THE PROTOCOL

To practice the protocol, first make sure you understand the deadly effect emotions have on the body, mind, and spirit. Motivate yourself not to continue the same path that is destroying your youthfulness.

Second, do daily meditations for at least 30 minutes before bed. Make sure to achieve ultra-stillness and emptiness, which are more important than the length of time. Usually when you start, it may take a long time to reach this "chi-gong state." After you practice for a while, you will be able to reach the chi-gong state immediately. The chi-gong state is more advanced than the state of mind we achieve when performing microcosmic orbit chi-gong presented in last chapter for energy balancing. This is because the latter requires mind concentration to the energy points and meridians. So it is still not entirely empty. Therefore, it is desirable that before you start practicing the protocols of this chapter you perform the energy balance work of the last chapter.

Third, set your mind and lifestyle so that you completely separate the two lives, the modern life and your true original nature. You must allocate as much time as possible to live the true life of your original nature.

Let's conclude by quoting the *Tao-De-Ching*, the second most printed book in the world (after the Bible), by Lao Tzu.

The five colors blind the eye,
The five tones deafen the ear,
The five flavors dull the taste,
Racing and hunting madden the mind,
Precious things lead one astray.

Therefore the sage is guided by what he feels and not by
    what he sees.
He lets go of that and chooses this.
Yield and overcome;
Bend and be straight;
Empty and be full;
Wear out and be new;
Have little and gain;
Have much and be confused.

Therefore wise men embrace the one
And set an example to all.
Not putting on a display,
They shine forth.

Not justifying themselves,
They are distinguished.
Not boasting,
They receive recognition.
Not bragging,
They never falter.
They do not quarrel,
So no one quarrels with them.

Therefore the ancients say, "Yield and overcome."
Is that an empty saying?
Be really whole,
And all things will come to you.[*]

---

[*] *Tao Te Ching*, Lao Tzu, translated by Gia-Fu Feng and Jane English, Vintage Books, New York, 1972.

CHAPTER 8

SIXTH PROTOCOL: REFINE SEXUAL ENERGY

As I was sitting on a big limestone stairway in front of a magnificent Taoist temple in south China, a mystic Taoist told me the story of He Shouwu. "You know, it is the name of this magic herb that all of us use. But it was named after a true person. There was an old fellow living in a small village. He could not get married because he was impotent, weak, and very poor. At age 54, he had a dream about taking a kind of grass root he'd seen high up in the mountains to restore his sexual vitality and transmute this newfound energy into long life. When he woke up, he went to fetch this root. He practiced the transmutation method and took the herbs.

"His hair turned black. His cheeks and lips turned red and opaque, full of vibrant light. He restored his sexual vitality. He was stronger than ever. He got married at age 59, had 6 children, and died at age 160."

"Very intriguing," I said. "How did he transmute the energy?"

"Well, life force, the energy which sustains life, is reflected through sexual vitality. It is limited. It is mostly leaked away through semen and blood throughout our lives.

It is like oil in a lamp that burns away. The learned ones know how to transmute the heat back to the oil so that the flame lasts forever."

"Can you teach me?" I asked, eager to know.

"Don't hurry. I'll teach you when you are ready. You must first build your foundation."

Standing up, we walked together toward the peak of the fog-covered mountains, deeply breathing the energetic, electrifying air.

My annual trip to China always makes me feel like a little child—knowing so little and being so curious with these sacred teachers. It keeps me coming back time after time.

Ping's Dairy

Can people really reach immortality? The ancients believed it could be done. Let us explain the meaning of immortality as they understood it. As mentioned, humans have three treasures, essence, chi, and spirit. When the spirit energy becomes very high and strong, it grows out of the physical body and elevates into the universe, becoming an immortal being. Therefore, when talking about immortality, we do not mean physical immortality.

As discussed, Taoists believe that everything in the universe is energy: plants, animals, rocks, mountains, oceans, etc. Humans consist of three levels of energy vibrating at different frequencies. The three levels correspond to the three treasures in humans—essence, chi, and spirit.

To review the human energy systems, the first level is the physical plane, comprised of flesh and bones and vital essence, such as enzymes, blood, semen, and body fluids. This is the first treasure, the essence. Everything on the physical plane is at an energy frequency that is mortal, following the law of entropy and the law of life. It will decay toward disorganization and degeneration. All we can hope is to preserve and prolong it.

The second level is the energy plane. When essence and spirit energy are strong, chi (energy) is vibrant. It sustains life, making it vibrant. This energy level is more subtle. It vibrates at a level between mortal and immortal. Chi is a very real phenomenon. It is largely not measurable by modern technology, but its existence has been demonstrated by many scientists.

The third level is the spiritual plane. Spirit energy is prenatal, existing before we are conceived. It is an energy that vibrates beyond the speed of light and possesses negative entropy, always moving toward organization. Combined with the parents' essence (sperm in the father and egg in the mother), the spirit conceives a new life. Mother's essence (blood) continues to nurture the embryo until birth. During our lifetime, this spirit energy can be depleted or increased. Through long-term emotional stress, we can easily deplete chi. The body has to make up the lost chi in order to sustain life, thus depleting essence and spirit energy. When spirit energy is reduced, not only is life weakened, but also we leave the world as a lower level of energy, becoming a lower level of being in the energy universe when we die. This is what the ancients meant by heaven and hell, god and ghosts. There are many things in between too.

We are born possessing a certain level of prenatal spirit energy. In the course of our lifetime, this very precious energy gradually grows weaker.

The purpose of Taoist alchemy is to refine postnatal essence into spirit energy, thus increasing our spirit energy potential. Through a lifetime of practice, we have the opportunity to dramatically strengthen the spirit energy, thus not only sustaining a very long young life but also elevating into higher beings, the immortals. When this happens, the physical body becomes irrelevant. Immortals can switch between physical bodies and subtle energies.

This explanation of immortality is beyond current sciences and technology. However, there have been observations of such energy transformation. One was reported in the authoritive book *I Ching and Traditional Chinese Medicine* by Dr. Yang Li. During a mission in May 1987, the Russian space shuttle encountered a strong set of "lights." It consisted of seven huge human-like objects with wings and foggy light rings. Appearing to be several hundred feet tall, they followed the shuttle for at least ten minutes and were recorded on video for 43 minutes. The Russian physicist Monagov said, "These things no doubt were some type of human-like beings. However, they have evolved into a stage so advanced that they can transition between physical bodies and a set of light clouds."

This event has raised many questions: Can human beings evolve into an advanced state where they can transition between different times and spaces instantaneously? How do all these different times and spaces relate to each other? After death, do their remains (spirit) transition to another time and space to continue to live? Under what conditions can they return to the human physical world? Some scientists postulate that the human genetics must be beyond four-dimensional time and space. After all, within seven weeks of growth, an embryo has repeated 300 million years of evolution. This process must be beyond our comprehension of time and space. It must be beyond the speed of light.

After all, we have immortals right with us. Our genes are immortal. They pass from generation to generation.

UNLEASHING OUR ENERGY CAPACITY

Most of the methods of this chapter will be based on chi-gong. Chi-gong is the best medium to condition our bodies and minds into the spiritual energy space. Once we can connect ourselves to this high level energy plane, we open ourselves to become a higher being, more spiritually developed, able to communicate to the immortal energy source of the universe, able to change between physical and spiritual planes any time we want, and ultimately able to become immortal and forever young. We may never get to the ultimate state of energy. But even just 10% of that is quite a reward for those who seek to stay younger longer and live in good health for more years.

Why is chi-gong able to create such miracles? Humans have a much larger innate capacity to live than we usually tap into. When a typical person dies, he or she has used only 20% of brain cells, 20% of microblood vessels, and 50% DNA capacity. The human body also has incredible metabolism, digestion, and heart muscle fiber capacity. This extra capacity can be used through chi-gong.

The human brain has two aspects, consciousness and subconsciousness. During billions of years of evolution, the subconscious mind is largely suppressed. We are a lot less intuitive than people were thousands of years ago. There are still people, the psychic ones, who can sense past and future, who help law enforcement search for criminals by their intuition rather than reasoning. Most of them would say they seem connected with a mysterious force or person that gives them signals. Some animals get very restless right before an earthquake. Some of us feel something strange happening when a relative dies or during other big events, happy or unhappy. Some of us even have dreams about future events. This is the working of the subconscious mind! Chi-gong is meant to explore the remaining 80% of our brain cells. It is believed this part of the brain, although never used, contains unawakened information, such as pre-life memories, space and time communication of past and future, sensing signals that most of us cannot perceive. Thus chi-gong can reverse evolution and unleash the vast power of the brain.

An interesting experiment was conducted by Dr. Justa Smith, a biochemist. She wondered if laying-on-hands healing could actually affect a body's enzyme system. You will recall that enzymes are the agents which activate all the body biochemical processes, i.e., metabolism. Different enzymes are targeted to different processes, such as digestive enzymes for decomposing food. Dr. Smith found that healers can either speed up activity for some types of enzymes or slow down others. Since healers did not know which enzymes govern which activities, the energy or chi that was passed to the enzymes by healers seemed to have some "intelligence," i.e., selectivity. Dr. Smith further studied a biochemistry flowchart to see where each of the "treated" enzymes fit into the normal pathways of cellular energy metabolism. She observed that the change of enzyme activity produced by the healers was always in the direction of greater energy reserve and increased health of the body's cells. Therefore, the healers' energy, or chi, knows exactly which enzymes to accelerate or decelerate.

As we discussed in Chapter 2, the human system, like other thermodynamic systems, follows the direction of the second law of thermodynamics. It possesses the property of positive entropy, always going from a more organized state to a less organized state. Entropy thus describes the aging process. Dr. Smith's experiments showed that the energy (or chi) imparted by healers possesses properties that reduce entropy because it always moved the system toward a more organized state. Some physicists call this property "negative entropy" or extropy. If a healer treats cancer, the enzymes which promote cancer growth are inhibited, while the enzymes which promote immune response are strengthened automatically. The exact mechanism of the human energy system is patently unclear to modern technology and sciences at their current level of understanding.

If through chi-gong we can achieve negative entropy, which is immortal by definition, our job becomes to use our body's resources during our lifetime to maximize the energy component in us, which possesses negative entropy. If we can do this as much as possible, we are cultivating the most negative entropy component of our total energy and we are closer to a true immortal.

To unleash the great power of the brain is to awaken and strengthen the spirit energy. It is similar to the alchemy process in chemistry. It requires raw materials to start with. In Taoist alchemy, sexual energy is the raw material from which great spirit energy is refined and stored.

What exactly are we preserving as life force energy? To be specific, we are preserving semen in males and menstrual blood in females. In fact, we want to preserve the prenatal and postnatal energy that will be used to create semen and blood. Men expend great energy through sexual intercourse, masturbation, and wet dreams. On the other hand, for women, it is mostly through blood loss in the menstrual period.

THE HUMAN SEXUAL ENERGY

One of the most potent energies that humans can produce is sexual energy. It is critical to health, longevity, and immortality— depending on how we use it. Unlike other potent energies created in us, sexual energy can be used for higher purposes of longevity and immortality. Other energy forms, such as enzymes, can only be preserved. They cannot be refined.

Scientists divide human life into three main stages: childhood (from birth to puberty); adulthood (able to reproduce); and senescence (post reproduction). As you can see, sex, or the ability to conceive, is a deciding factor in each stage of life.

The first stage is also called the extropy stage. This is because it possesses the property of negative entropy, always moving toward more organization. This scientific classification is consistent with the ancient law of life discussed in Chapter 2. The second stage is called the plateau phase. In this phase, we gradually release energy (limited potential) to sustain life, so our life is gradually washed away. The third stage is the rapid descent phase, in which life quickly degenerates—the maximum rate of entropy toward disorganization.

Puberty is a very important milestone in life. Puberty usually begins around age 15 for boys and 13 for girls. For males, signs of puberty include development of hair around the penis and testicles, increase in penis size, descending and increased size of testicles, hair under the arms, facial hair, hair on the lower stomach, deepening of the voice, possible voice cracking (inconsistent high-pitched tone in the voice), possible chest hair, increase in height, libido development (increased interest or drive for sex or stimulation of the penis), possible increase in facial oils, possible acne, the ability to produce sperm and semen, and the ability to fertilize a female's egg through sexual intercourse.

For females, signs are development of breasts and hips, beginning of a monthly menstrual period (ovulation cycle and bleeding from the uterus/vaginal area), possible heightened tone of voice, development of hair around the vagina and underarms, possible minor facial hair, increase in height, libido development (increased interest or drive for sex or stimulation of the vagina), possible increase in facial oils, possible acne, and the ability to become pregnant through sexual intercourse with a male. In general, for both sexes, the ultimate criterion is the ability to reproduce offspring.

Puberty is the start of sexual energy maturity and also the period when sex hormones peak. As discussed in the law of life in Chapter 2, the I Ching hexagram of the life cycle indicates peak energy at around age 14 for females and 16 for males. From this point on, life drains away through spirit energy loss and vital essence loss.

How correct were our ancient sages? It is interesting to note the statistics on mortality rates in the U.S. in 1976, data compiled by Gee EM, Veevers, et al, titled "Accelerating sex differentials in mortality: an analysis of contributing factors," published in *Social Biology* in 1984. In that data, the white mortality rate starts at around 1,500 per 100,000 population at birth. It drops gradually to the lowest point around age 15 to approximately 25 per 100,000 for females and 40 per 100,000 for males. From this point on, it increases dramatically over time as we age.

You may think that age 25 is the strongest age. But from both ancient and current statistics, age 25 is inferior to age 15. The mortality rate at 25 reported in the same data shows about 60 per 100,000 for females and 160 for males, far higher than at age 15. By age 40, the rate increases to around 150 per 100,000 for females and 250 for males. Therefore, *a healthy delay of puberty prolongs life span.*

It is also interesting to note that the "ability to reproduce" (puberty) signals the start of the decline of life. Somehow, the activity of reproduction (or sex) has to pay a price, a price of burning our life candles, reducing our health and longevity. There seem to be extreme cases in nature which amplify this observation. For example, certain worms, fruit flies, and pacific salmon all die immediately after reproductive activities. It seems that the purpose of their life is to reproduce. After that, they become useless and are supposed to die. Others die gradually after reproductive activities. This is true for most mammals.

Reproductive activities are very costly to life. In Taoist alchemy, it is believed that sperm in men and blood (during menstrual period) in women are produced by converting some of the body's most precious prenatal and postnatal vital essence. They also consume the precious chi. Therefore, it is a major cost to health and longevity to reproduce offspring or engage in frequent leakage of semen or a large amount of blood during menstrual periods in women. Ancient sages believed that one drop of semen equaled one hundred drops of blood.

According to the evolutionary life history theory, one of the modern theories of aging, natural selection for the clock genes—those which dictate the onset (puberty) and duration (menopause) of the period of maximum fertility and reproductive competence—directly impacts potential life span. The earlier you achieve your puberty (maturation of reproductivity) and the quicker you consume all your reproductive reservoir (semen and blood), the faster you age. In evolution, natural selection has put the time clock in our genes that favors the ones who are still useful to maximize the production of offspring. The less the ability still remaining to reproduce, the quicker the "aging" clock runs. In general, it is a price we pay for accelerated puberty and accelerated leakage of semen and blood.

In nature, semen is supposed to be expended only at mating season. Nature also only allows the strongest and most fit males to perform sexual activities. The weak and old are not able to put up the fight. This is the natural selection of evolution—only the best seeds reproduce offspring. Thus through natural selection, living things evolve to a more advanced level and survive for millions of years.

From a modern medical viewpoint, semen consists of a mixture of sperm from the testicles and fluid from the seminal vesicles and prostate gland, but it also contains smaller amounts of other fluids secreted from glands along the urethra. Sixty percent of semen comes from glands called the seminal vesicles, whereas 38% comes from the prostate, with the remainder from other glands. The prostate contribution is responsible for the characteristic odor. The fluid from the seminal vesicles is high in fructose, a type of naturally occurring sugar, which provides primary nourishment for the traveling sperm. Semen contains vitamins, minerals, trace elements, hormones, proteins, ions, als, trace elements, hormones, proteins, ions, enzymes, and other vital nutritional substances. From a purely chemical point of view, it appears inconsequential to lose semen. However, what modern technology cannot measure is the chi that is involved in the generation of semen. This chi is related to life and death.

Thus, reducing leakage of semen (in males) and menstrual blood (in females) increases life span and delays aging.

Charlie Chaplin wrote in his autobiography, "Like Balzac, who believed that a night of sex meant the loss of a good page of his novel, so I believed that it meant the loss of a good day's work at the studio."

There was an interesting dialog in the April 1975 issue of *Playboy* magazine with jazz musician Miles Davis:

Davis: You can't come, then fight or play. You can't do it. When I get ready to come, I come. But I do not come and play.

Interviewer: Explain that in layman's terms.

Davis: Ask Muhammad Ali. If he comes, he can't fight two minutes. Shit, he couldn't even whip me.

Interviewer: Would you fight Muhammad Ali under those conditions, to prove your point?
Davis: You're goddam right I'd fight him. But he's got to promise to fuck first. If he ain't going to fuck, I ain't going to fight. You give up all your energy when you come. I mean, you give up all of it! So, if you're going to fuck before a gig, how are you going to give something when it's time to hit?

If we think about it, many people experience tiredness after frequent leakage of semen or around the time of the menstrual period. We tend to catch cold easily and want some rest. Some people even use this as a kind of "sleeping pill."

In summary, sexual energy— semen (in male) and blood (or egg and menstrual blood in female)—is the most potent energy humans can produce. The entire human aging process is timed through stages of sexuality. Life expectancy is based on the timing of puberty and the speed that sexual energy is drained. Preserving and refining sexual energy increases longevity and immortality.

ACCELERATED ENERGY DEPLETION

In modern societies, we accelerate nature's course in the leaking of our vital essence. Overnutrition has speeded up the start of puberty. Sex is a large part of the economy. Motivated by profit, many businesses, in the adult, fashion, and entertainment industries, for example, work hard to overstimulate sexual activities and arousals, accelerating the leaking of sexual essence and resulting in earlier aging.

Citing an article in the October 18, 1999 issue of *Newsweek* magazine, "According to a study published this month in the journal *Pediatrics*, most white girls show signs of puberty before the age of 10, compared with about 15 at the turn of the 20th century. There are indications that some kids—especially in low-income inner-city neighborhoods—are also becoming sexually active at an alarmingly early age. According to a 1997 Centers for Disease Control study, 6.5 percent of ninth-grade girls—compared with only 2.9 percent of 12th graders—said they had had sex before the age of 13. Boys showed a similar increase: 14.7 percent of ninth graders said they'd already been sexually active, while only 6 percent of 12th graders said they'd had sex before the age of 13."

According to the book *Sex in America*, by Robert Michael, et al., based on the 1992 University of Chicago study conducted by the National Health and Social Life Survey, "The average age of first sexual intercourse for women has been reduced from about 19 for people who were born in the 1930's down to 17.5 for those born in the 1960's. The same holds true for men. The first intercourse for men has been reduced from 18 for those born in the 1930's to 17 for those born in the 1960's."

Similar data was reported in a Durex Global Sex Survey in 1997. Here are some of the findings about the age of first intercourse and frequency of intercourse:

The trend toward having sex at a younger age is accelerating with each decade. Respondents over 40 reported their first sexual experience at an average age of 18.6 years, compared to an average age of 18 years for 30-39 year-olds. Americans are the youngest to start having sex with an average of 16.2 years. People in Hong Kong (18.9 years) and Poland (18.7) wait the longest to have their first sexual experience.

The global average for frequency of intercourse among respondents is 2.1 times per week. Americans lead with 2.6 times per week, or 24% higher than the average. People from Thailand have the lowest average sexual frequency at 1.2 times per week. The most sexually active age ranges are the 20-29 and 30-39 year-olds.

According to a number of studies, many post-pubescent young men report daily ejaculation, if not more frequently than that. This frequency gradually declines for most males to 2-3 time per week, which is typical of men in their forties.

According to the 1992 University of Chicago National Health and Social Life Survey, on the average, 15% of men masturbate (of course, to ejaculation) once a week.

Thus, our sexual energy is overtaxed in modern society, typified by earlier puberty and more expenditure of sexual fluids (semen and blood), leading to accelerated aging and degenerative diseases.

SEXUAL PLEASURE, ORGASM, AND EJACULATION

You may ask, isn't it a natural process for males to leak semen and females to leak blood? Isn't it nature's design to program life's clock to gradually consume life energy toward death? It is the law of life and the entropy of life.

What can we do about it? Does preserving sexual energy mean reducing sexual pleasure?   We cannot control nature's course. After all, sex in humans is not just a reproductive activity; it is also for enjoyment. How can we avoid it? Besides, there is no way to change a woman's menstrual period.

In fact, we are able to change this natural process and simultaneously increase enjoyment. The purpose in doing so is to refine and transmute our sexual energy (the raw materials) to the spirit energy, leading to extended young life, longevity, and immortality. This reverses nature's course. There is an old Taoist saying, "For death, follow the flow of life; for life, reverse the flow of life."

In the Chinese classic *Secret of the Jade Bedroom*, there is a dialog between the Yellow Emperor's two counselors, held 5,000 years ago:

Rainbow girl: It is generally assumed that a man gains great pleasure from ejaculation. But when he learns the Tao of yin and yang, he will ejaculate less and less. Will this not diminish his pleasure as well?

Peng Tze: Not at all! After ejaculation, a man feels tired, his ears buzz, his eyes get heavy, and he longs for sleep. He is thirsty and his limbs feel weak and stiff. By ejaculating, he enjoys a brief moment of sensation, but suffers long hours of weariness as a result. This is no true pleasure!

However, if a man regulates his ejaculation to an absolute minimum and retains his semen, his body will grow strong, his mind will be clear, and his vision and hearing will improve. Is preserving sexual energy meant to reduce sexual pleasure?

To appreciate this, we need to understand the difference between orgasm and ejaculation. *What is the difference between having five ejaculations (and thus five orgasms) a week as compared with five orgasms a day without ever ejaculating? The level of pleasure of the latter is 100 times higher!* The pleasure to a partner is also immense because females usually require a longer time to reach orgasms and they desire more frequent orgasms.

An important project in the 1950's was performed by Dr. John C. Lilly through neurological studies of monkeys. He discovered different points in the brain that control the sexual response of male monkeys.

Dr. Lilly found that the neural points are different for different sexual functions. One neural point regulates arousal (erection). A second point regulates the orgasm itself (sensation of sexual peak and bliss of maximal satisfaction). The third point regulates muscular contraction (ejaculation).

The first and the second neural points control the pleasure, or entertainment aspects of sexual activities. The third one controls the reproductive aspect, of sexual activity, i.e., ejaculation of sperm to give new life. In the usual course of life, we combine all three activities as though they have to go together. Thus we limit ourselves in the enjoyment (because we cannot continuously ejaculate) and we pay the price of expending chi to build the potent semen.

Other research also indicates that stimulation of the septum, a portion of the brain known to be a part of the limbic system, results in the feeling of an orgasm, but this stimulation produces neither an erection nor ejaculation. These findings support the theory that ejaculation and orgasm, though often linked together, are, indeed, separate events.

Besides neurology of the brain, is there any other evidence, in layman's terms that this separation of pleasure (erection and orgasm) and reproduction (ejaculation) is meaningful?   A 1992 National Health and Social Life Survey discovered that only 29% of women always have orgasms and 75% of men always have orgasms (and ejaculations). On the other hand, about 40% of both men and women said they are extremely satisfied with their sexual intercourse emotionally.   Thus ejaculation and pleasure from sex are not all the same. They are controlled by different parts of the brain.

Although Lilly did not try to apply this research to human beings, his discovery indicates that *it is possible, through conscious and learned control, for us to completely separate the entrainment center of the process of erection (circulatory system) and orgasm (neural system) from the mechanics of ejaculation (muscular system).   If we can separate the two purposes of sexual activity, we can indeed maximize pleasure and minimize aging.*

Are men and women happy about their sexual life? The July/August 1999 issue of *Men's Health* reported a survey of 100 polygraphed women. It was found that 91% of women fake orgasms.   The remaining 9% said no, they never fake orgasms…well, maybe once in awhile.   Some 63% of women want sex to last longer, and the same amount want more frequent sex. Apparently, men need to last longer to get women more satisfied.

Are men happy about modern sex life? Not necessarily. Through the accelerated use of sexual energy, men quickly discharge their vitality and become old and impotent sooner. In the last dynasty of China, the Ching Dynasty, several generations of kings died young because one of the fashions of the palace was to surround the kings with dozens of wives and concubines. The kings indulged in unlimited sex, music, and food. They could not sustain their lives long because they consumed their vital essence much too quickly.

Are you surprised at the popularity of Viagra? According to *Yahoo Health*, the definition of impotence is: "The inability to achieve and maintain penile erection sufficient to complete satisfactory intercourse." They said that occasional impotence occurs "in about half of adult men in the U.S.; chronic impotence affects about one in eight American men."

Yahoo Health listed the following causes of impotence:
- Medication use (especially antihypertensives)
- Smoking
- Hormonal deficiency caused by disease (diabetes) or injury
- Liver disease, usually caused by alcoholism
- Circulation problems (arteriosclerosis, anemia, or vascular surgery)
- Neurological problems (injury, trauma, disease)
- Urological procedures (prostatectomy, orchiectomy, radiation therapy)
- Penile implants (or prostheses) that function improperly
- Depression, anxiety, fatigue, boredom, stress, fear of failure
- Mood-altering drugs, alcohol, medications
- Fear of infection

- Fear of recurring heart problems
- Deep-seated psychological problems

Note that the important thing not listed here is the deterioration of general vitality due to overleakage of vital essence. In general, the fundamental reason for impotence is because of the accelerated aging effect as a result of vital life force drainage.

Since leakage of semen is a bad thing, what about people who do not have interest in sex and masturbation? Are they necessarily more healthy? The answer is no. First of all, they cannot escape the involuntary semen leakage through wet dreams, which average once a week for young men and once a month for middle-age men. Second, there is some significant benefit from an active stimulation of sexual hormones. Growth hormone (HGH) in your body (not administrated externally) is a vital hormone which stimulates growth, repair, the immune system, muscle building, bone health, skin elasticity, and cartilage strength. It is called the hormone of youth. It is well known that sex steroids greatly stimulate the pituitary gland, which in turn secretes growth hormones. In the book *Grow Young with HGH* by Dr. Ronald Klatz, 1997, it was stated, "Testosterone is a strong growth hormone stimulant. Several studies have found that testosterone replacement in men who are deficient raised their levels of growth hormone and IGF-1.

"In 1993, a team of researchers led by Curtis J. Hobbs of the Madigan Army Medical Center in Tacoma, Washington, found that when men with normal levels of male sex hormones were given testosterone, their IGF-1 levels rose from an average of 293.5 nanograms per milliliter to 354.9 nanograms per milliliter— putting them at a high functioning level." The rise in IGF-1 levels, the author suggests, "might serve as a mechanism for several observed effects of T (testosterone). These include improvements in osteoporosis and body building."

Therefore, active sexual life is very important to the vitality of life. Please understand that when we talk about the benefit of HGH and testosterone, we refer to the ones generated by your own body, rather than externally injected or orally taken. It is unfortunate that people have to risk having these hormones replaced. Wouldn't it be nice to have vibrant health, plenty of HGH and testosterone for a long period of your life, say 150 years, without the need of seeking solutions with unknown risks? Let's improve ourselves naturally using our own innate ability.

In conclusion, sexual energy is the most potent energy humans can produce, but it is very easy to leak the energy and deplete life. It needs to be preserved to prolong youth and life. Sex can kill you or make you immortal. It depends on knowing how to preserve your energy! Orgasms and ejaculations can be separated. Ejaculation is nature's design to reproduce. Natural selection diminishes the usefulness of the living things which have done their job for reproduction and thus starts to accelerate the aging clock and degeneration. Orgasms, without ejaculation, can not only stimulate hormones to invigorate the whole body energy system and to create 100 times more enjoyment of life through sex, but can liberate the sexual energy for potential refinement through Taoist alchemy to higher energy, which ultimately leads to the path of immortality.

APPLYING THE PROTOCOL

Taoist Seminal Alchemy is a very deep practice that few can learn from books. It has to be taught directly from real teachers face-to-face. We do not intend to cover this topic in depth but to provide some elementary practices beneficial to health and longevity.

We would like to introduce several techniques for preserving and refining sexual energy. Some apply to men only, others to both male and female. For men, the first objective is to have many orgasms without ejaculations. Sometimes this is called valley orgasms because you reach peak sexual bliss or excitement many times and still retain the ability for continued intercourse.

The second objective is to transmute the aroused sexual energy to higher spirit energy. For women, the objective is to reduce or stop the loss of menstrual blood and transmute the sexual energy to spirit energy. The methods we present here are: the "emergency measure" of Huiyin lock (for men only); the Huiyin draw method (for men only); the microcosmic orbit circulation of vital essence method (for both men and women), and the chi-gong state method (for both men and women). They are in the order of increasing difficulty of practice.

The "Emergency Measure" of Huiyin Lock

This is a basic method for men only. When you first practice the techniques of this chapter, you may not be able to control the timing of the peak orgasm point. You may pass the point and move into ejaculation. There is a method you can use to save most of your precious semen and half of the energy expenditure.

At ejaculation, sperm and testis fluid travel in a tiny tube through the prostate. At the prostate, it mixes with the fluid secreted from the prostate. Together the combined fluid or semen is ejaculated through the urethra through the penis. The fluid passes through the perineum between the anus and the penis, also known as the root of the penis, or Huiyin energy center (the gate of life). As part of the penis, Huiyin is usually soft, but turns hard as the penis becomes erect.

An effective way to stop the leak at ejaculation is to use both hands to press the Huiyin point. Once Huiyin is pressed, semen can not come out at ejaculation. In the meantime, the body continues through all the motion, emotion, and feeling of ejaculation.

This is not the optimal method, though, because you still lose some energy. The semen trapped in the portion of the tubes above Huiyin will be expelled during urination. There is also associated energy at ejaculation that will be lost. However, it is better than the total loss of semen in the usual way of ejaculation. You won't feel as tired with Huiyin lock as you do with the usual ejaculation.

The Huiyin Draw Method

Huiyin draw method is similar to the Huiyin lock method, except, instead of using hands, you use mind, breath, and muscle around the Huiyin center. It must be used before ejaculation is inevitable. At the brink of ejaculation, use the mind to draw a deep breath in from Huiyin upward into Tan Tien (inside the navel). In the meantime, contract the muscle around Huiyin to help pull it upward. Do this several times until the severe urge subsides.

Microcosmic Orbit Energy Refinement

The purpose of this method is to refine the potent sexual energy into higher spiritual energy. Sexual energy is excited during several different activities: men's morning involuntary erection, wet dreams, sexual intercourse, masturbation and other arousals for both men and women, and a woman's menstrual period.

For men, the morning involuntary erection is the most potent sexual energy. It is untamed by desire and craving of the mind. It is nature's design of the most natural energy peak cycle. All men have a daily cycle of testosterone levels that peak somewhere between 4 and 6 a.m. This coincides with the time when many men have early morning erections. These involuntary erections are a normal part of the sleep cycle for most men and, according to research, most men have perhaps three or four each night. There are various theories as to why nature planned it this way. One suggests that this is a way the male penis "renews" itself with an ample supply of oxygen.

In the celebrated I Ching, the ancient sages divided the energy cycle of each day according to the waxing and waning of yin and yang energies. Between 9 to 11 p.m. is the extreme of yin energy. Yang energy starts to emerge between 11 p.m. to 1 a.m., and reaches its maximum between 7 to 9 a.m. Therefore Taoists believe the early morning erection corresponds to the peak yang energy in the body. If sexual energy is the most potent energy, its peak is even more potent. We must take advantage of this peak energy as the raw materials to refine into higher energy.

In the early years of post-pubescence, nighttime erections are frequently accompanied by full-fledged ejaculations. Wet dreams gradually occur less frequently as men grow older, and masturbation and sexual intercourse become increasingly important. We want to prevent such leakage of semen during wet dreams.

Taoists believe that before birth in the mother's womb, yin and yang are united. The spirit, an energy, enters the life (made of mother and father's vital essence) through the opening on top of the head. Life in the prenatal stage is well balanced. At birth, upon the first lung breaths, life is separated from the original nature. Yin and yang are separated. Yin energy sinks down to the kidney, yang energy (pertaining to the mind) goes up to the heart, and spirit is housed inside the Niwuan cavity behind the midpoint of the eyebrows. Once yin and yang are separated, they will gradually be out of balance due to the leakage of vital essence and spirit energy.

The purpose of the Taoist alchemy is to return us to the state of the womb, uniting yin and yang. When the original yin is stirred when our sexual energies are naturally aroused, it is vital to circulate this energy upwards to let it unite with the yang energy, i.e., the heart and the spirit.

In Chinese, *Tan* means "elixir" and *Tien* means "field." Elixir in Taoist alchemy means a highly refined concentrated form of immortal energy. Once such energy is refined, one can reach immortality.

Man has three Tan Tiens: the lower Tan Tien inside the naval where the prenatal vital essence is housed; the middle Tan Tien midway between the naval and the midpoint of the nipples, where the prenatal chi is stored; and the upper Tan Tien between the eyebrows and approximately one-third into the head, where the original spirit is housed.

The full extent of Taoist alchemy runs very deep and far. It is impossible to cover it all here. You should keep in mind, however, that yin energy accumulated from the stirring of the sexual essence can be vaporized through meditation and drawn upward into middle and upper Tan Tiens, where the yin energy, or sexual essence, copulates with the yang energy of the original chi and spirit and they are upgraded into higher energy. When this energy becomes large and dense, it becomes the elixir of immortality.

In men, the potent sexual essence is excited in the following scenarios: in the morning, when the penis is erect naturally, without thought; at night, when the penis is erect during sleep; and during sexual intercourse and masturbation.

Use the microcosmic orbit refinement to circulate such energy through the Du and Ren meridians:

During sexual excitement, breathe in to draw the yin energy from Huiyin up through the Du meridian all the way to the crown (the top of the head), then breathe out to drive the energy down through Ren meridian back to the lower Tan Tien. This way, the concentrated sexual yin energy is mixed with yang energy in the upper energy centers. Yin and yang copulate to become more refined energies. Wet dreams are quite unconscious events. Most of the time when we wake up it is too late. Therefore, if you have a history of frequent wet dreams, you should perform microcosmic orbit chi-gong before sleep to calm the mind and energy and thus prevent the leakage.

For women, it is a little bit different. The main leakage occurs during the monthly menstrual period. During ovulation, prenatal and postnatal energies are stimulated by the associated hormones. The ovaries function under the control of the pituitary gland in the head. The pituitary first makes a hormone which stimulates follicle growth and egg production, at the same time bringing about secretion of the hormone estrogen. Under estrogen influence the lining of the uterus thickens in preparation for receiving a fertilized egg. Then the hormone progesterone is produced. If the egg is not fertilized, progesterone production is halted and the lining of the uterus is shed at the monthly menstrual period. Thus the cycle starts again for the next month.

Taoists believe that this reproduction cycle requires significant energy expenditure, just as the release of semen does in men. Thus, absorbing such energy and refining it into higher energy becomes the goal for women.

A few days before the menstrual period, there will be signs of energy excitement. Usually women feel restless, dizzy, tired, or drowsy and have low back and leg soreness, swollen breasts, loss of appetite, or a heavy feeling in the lower abdominal area. Different people have different feelings. This is the time women need to meditate.

Women also have three Tan Tiens: upper Tan Tien of Tan-zhong midpoint between the nipples; middle Tan Tien, inside the navel; and lower Tan Tien, between the pubic bone and the navel corresponding to the ovaries.

A few days before the menstrual period, use the microcos-mic orbit chi-gong:

Calm the mind, close the eyes. Lightly focus (notice) on the Tanzhong cavity. Use both hands to smoothly massage the breasts. Inhale from the lower female Tan Tien (ovaries) down to Huiyin (between anus and vagina) and up through the Du meridian to the top of the head (the crown), then ex-hale down Ren meridian (middle line through front of body) to the upper female Tan Tien (midway between the nipples).

Once chi is full at the upper Tan Tien (warmness, etc.), move down to middle Tan Tien at the naval. Store chi at this point.

Repeat the exercise for half an hour.

You will notice that as you practice this meditation, bleed-ing during your period will lessen. In ancient Taoist alchemy, the goal is to return men and women to a pre-pubescent state. You will find your breasts become like a teenager's and your bleeding is slight. If you achieve this level of practice in middle age, you may delay or never experience menopause. For post-menopausal women, you should first practice microcosmic chi-gong until you regather enough chi to restart the monthly menstrual period. Then you can follow the method presented in this chapter to refine the energy.

Chi-gong State Method

This method applies to both men and women.

The chi-gong state is a particular state of body, mind, and spirit.   It is a level of total realization of subconsciousness, bliss, ultra-stillness, and emptiness. In such a state you are totally dissolved into the vast energy field of the universe. It is difficult to talk about the exact feeling in such a state because it is different for different people. Once you are trained and developed enough, you will know when you achieve such a chi-gong state.

To reach the fullness of the chi-gong state, you also need to practice the chi-gong methods already discussed. After you acquire some proficiency, you can easily initiate such a state by starting the chi-gong breathing. Recall that chi-gong breathing requires very slow, light, long breaths in and out continuously without the thought of breathing.   Start breathing into the belly (Tan Tien), gradually fill up the entire lungs, and breathe out, first emptying the lungs and then the belly. Ultimately, you will feel your whole body breathing. Once in this state, you will realize that you are not just breathing air but you are also breathing energy through all the large and small meridians and channels in communication with the surrounding energies from the environment.

During sex, or before sleep, or at dawn when your penis is erect, or before the menstrual period, you can achieve a state of bliss by initiating chi-gong breathing. You can increase dramatically the length of sexual intercourse before ejaculation. Furthermore, if both partners perform chi-gong breathing during sexual intercourse, there is a maximum energy exchange between them, especially when the partners are of different sex, thus yin (female) and yang (male) energies are maximally copulated. This is a great benefit to health and longevity because yin needs yang, and yang requires yin. It helps balance the body energy.

To help you appreciate the effect that chi-gong can exert on the internal energy systems, organs, and hormonal and nervous systems, we want to talk about an interesting experiment. It is reported in the pioneering book *Creating Energy Body Sciences* by the famous Chinese physicist Qian Xue San, published in 1989. Scientist and chi-gong master Wang Ja Lin of the Yuanang Human Chi-gong Research Institute of China allowed his own gallbladder to be wired to all sorts of instruments for four months' observation. The experiment compared the physiology among the chi-gong state, the relaxed state, and sleeping state. It was found that in the chi-gong state, secretion from the gallbladder is much higher than the usual rest and sleep states, demonstrating that chi-gong indeed can dramatically alter the course of life. Many other reports show that chi-gong can affect the recovery of muscle strains and change heart rates.

Therefore, we use the chi-gong state to stimulate hormones and to enjoy sex without leakage of semen and blood. This higher practice allows us to stop using the mind to think about anything, including the entertainment of sex activities. The mind is withdrawn. Body, mind, and spirit become one. Anything physical, including thought, is empty and gone. You are totally dissolved into the macrocosm of the universe. A selective turn on and off of this state during sexual activities is particularly rewarding but requires higher training. In the advanced state of alchemy, although your essence, chi, and spirit energies are full, you do not have the craving for indulgence in sex.

This chapter has only scratched the surface of Taoist alchemy. It is an endless learning process. Advanced practice, difficult to explain in a book, requires face-to-face teachings from a real master. No matter how trained you are, you will always be a student of a practice so deep and so mystical.

CHAPTER 9

SEVENTH PROTOCOL: REVERSE THE EFFECTS OF GRAVITY

Dr. Smith, a space medicine doctor, was sitting across from me, the second time he had visited my office. As we finished up the treatment, I said curiously, "If people could spend years in space, would they live longer?"

"Longevity in space is not well studied. In space medicine, we mainly study the physiology of human response to changes of gravity, especially in a zero gravity situation."

Dr. Smith continued, thinking he had not quite satisfied my curiosity, "Since people have a lower metabolic rate living in a weightless environment (as compared to earth), they live slower. They must be able to live a lot longer, just like bears in hibernation."

"I agree. Just think about the ocean. Most ocean mammals are ageless. Animals like sharks, turtles, and rockfish, don't show signs of aging even when they are over 100 years old. They die because of predators and natural disasters. They also live in a near zero gravity environment in salt water."

Our living in a weightless environment is neither practical nor desirable. But what if we can come up with a therapy that reverses the impact of gravity on aging? We would be able to stay young longer.

Ping's Dairy

Taoist alchemy not only practices the preservation of vital essence and spirit energy, but it also believes in reversing life processes. Life is like an oil lamp. You can preserve it by burning it less and more efficiently, and you can also add oil. The adding oil process is called the reversal of life because life may get younger as more oil is added. For example, the last chapter talked about reversing life through sexual energy transmutation. Life's normal course is to leak away sexual energy through semen and blood. The purpose of sexual chi-gong is not only to preserve sexual essence but also to reverse the process by redirecting sexual energy upward to nourish the whole body, as opposed to letting it leak downward. In this protocol, the purpose is to reverse the negative impact of gravity. It is, in effect, reversing some aspect of evolution.

Billions of years of evolution have seen mankind go from living in the water to living on land. We now stand on two legs instead of four because our bodies have adjusted to the effect of the constant pulling down of gravity. Standing upright frees our hands to do many advanced things that other creatures cannot. However, there is a price to pay. The constant force of gravity pulling us down deteriorates our health over a long period.

Can we get the benefit of both the evolved and the unevolved? This chapter presents our last protocol of longevity. Again, due to the nature of the practice, it is difficult to learn without face-to-face assistance from learned teachers. We will only present the theory and elementary practice.

BODY UNDER GRAVITY

What is gravity, or g-force? Galileo was probably the first to look closely at the way objects fell to Earth. Legend has it that he climbed to the top of the leaning tower of Pisa and from there simultaneously dropped heavy and light balls, noting that they hit the ground at the same time. He thus demonstrated, contrary to some ancient claims, that heavy and light objects fell at the same rate.

A dropped object starts its fall quite slowly, but then steadily increases velocity. The velocity of a ball dropped from a high place increases each second by a constant amount, usually denoted by the small letter "g" (for gravity). The number for g, usually called the acceleration factor of gravity, is approximately 9.8. Thus, influenced by gravity, an object drops at a speed which increases by 9.8 meters per second.

Following Galileo, Isaac Newton continued the study of force. Among his many great discoveries, Newton learned the relationship among the force F which acts on an object, the mass M of the object, and its acceleration factor a (in the case of gravity, a is the same as g). In his celebrated first law of motion, the relationship is described by the following formula: $F = Ma$, or $F = Mg$ in the case of gravity.

Gravity, or g-force, is the large force acting upon us, which equals our weight. Think about this force pulling down the heart, liver, stomach, blood in the vessels, lymph fluids, etc. Luckily, we have all kinds of tissues pulling our organs up in place and our heart pumping blood upward to supply the brain and the upper extremities. However, for a 50-year-old person, he or she has been under this force for 50 years, constantly. When we stand straight up, all our vertical structures are especially effected by such a force. Our spines are pulled down, compressed, and grinded as we move under such force. No wonder we become shorter as we age;

all our bones are compressed at the discs and joints. Our organs, too, are pulled down as we age. The lower abdomen becomes larger, even without added fat.

We often hear about people having lowered stomachs. This is because the mechanisms for holding the organs in place (muscles, tendons, ligaments, and other membranes) are pulled and stretched over many years. Gravity pulls body fat downward as we age. We grow eye bags and double chins as the fat is pulled downward. More fat is pulled to the belly, hips, and thighs. Gravity also makes the buttocks and breasts sag. When we notice that everything is a half inch lower, we feel the impact of aging. Furthermore, our blood is pulled down too. When our heart is strong, this is okay. However, as the heart weakens with age, its ability to counter gravity by pumping blood up to the head and other small vessels in the upper parts of the body is less. Thus, the heart is more stressed, and the head is less nourished by blood. Gravity also increases metabolic rates, since the body has to counter the g-force.

Can we do away with gravity? No. We cannot live without gravity. Each part of us, through billions of years of evolution since our non-human ancestors climbed out of the ocean, has adapted to gravity. During short gravity free periods, we can temporarily lose our ability to fight gravity. A person on bed rest for too long can easily faint when he stands up because he loses his ability to withstand the g-force.

Man co-exists with gravity; without it, we simply cannot live. But gravity is also part of nature's law (the law of life) that wears us down. Do we accept it, or can we do something to lessen the negative impact?

Our blood system has adapted to vertical gravity. We are able to maintain an adequate supply of blood to the brain in the upright posture despite the heart having to pump the blood upward against gravity. This is made possible by certain compensatory mechanisms, which cause the small blood vessels in the legs to constrict, thus preventing the blood from pooling down. Our body has sensory mechanisms in the right heart ventricle. If the blood volume is low due to blood pulled down by g-force, several hormones, including rennin, aldosterone, and catecholamines, kick into action to stimulate a contraction of peripheral blood vessels, such as the ones in the legs. The contraction creates a narrower path for the blood downward and higher resistance (or blood pressure), thus making more blood available for the head.

Staying only a few days in a weightless environment or simply bed rest, results in biological deterioration. This is called a sub-g environment. Under such conditions, the vascular systems in the lower extremities do not need to restrict blood since there is no downward pulling by the g-force. After a while, you temporarily lose the capability. A sudden return to normal gravity—such as a space shuttle reentry, or sitting up after a long-term bed rest—may cause fainting because blood cannot be effectively restricted from pouring downwards. The brain does not have a sufficient supply of oxygen and glucose carried by blood. On the other hand, life in a hyper-gravity environment, such as may be experienced on a planet with 1.5 times the earth's gravity, would be miserable; we would have to lie down all the time due to an insufficient supply of blood to the head if we straightened up. It would also increase the evolutionary rate of development of bipedalism so that our lower blood vessels can restrict more.

The sub-g and hyper-g situation can be easily felt on an airplane ride. Remember your last flight? At takeoff, as the plane ascends, we experience a force more than the normal g, a hyper-g situation, because we are traveling opposite of the g-force. Our body is adapted to the normal g. When we are experiencing higher g's, our usual blood restriction mechanism is not sufficient. Therefore, we feel a temporary shortage of oxygen supply to the head: a faint feeling. To combat the additional g-force, our heart has to pump more blood to sustain the requirements of the brain. This in turn requires a higher metabolic rate and higher energy consumption. We can also feel the higher g-force drag our organs down lower than normal. Our muscles and ligaments are stretched further in order to hold the organs in place. These are some reasons that we tire easily after a flight.

As our plane descends, we experience a g-force which is a fraction of the usual because we are dropping in the same direction of gravity. Our head is now rushed with blood and our organs are suspended upward. To respond to this, our heart slows down and pumps less blood to the head. Our metabolic rate slows down too.

Flight just amplifies our sensation that something abnormal has happened to our physiology and autonomous control systems. On the ground, we are so used to the normal g-force that we don't even think of it. We forget about the force exerted on us every minute, every day of our lives.

Much of our life is about fighting gravity. Why does the heart pump harder when we run than when sitting still? It is because we fight harder against gravity.

Dr. Esar Shvartz presented a series of scientific experiments in his book *Biogravics*. It was shown that immersion in water produced a heart rate of 50, as compared to 60 for a recumbent position, 70 for a sitting position, 80 for standing, 110 for walking, and 140 for running. As gravity increases, our heart has to pump harder to supply blood to upper extremities. Being immersed in water is the easiest. We do not need to fight against gravity, largely because water provides the counteractive force to balance off gravity. It usually makes us very relaxed.

Sitting, standing and walking represent three other states. In a recumbent position, no attempt is made to oppose gravity except for the semiconscious metabolic functions. In sitting, an attempt is made to emerge from this condition. Man can maintain a sitting position for several hours, even though it requires substantial adjustments with respect to weight distribution, balance, and blood pooling. Some people who suffer from low blood pressure have difficulty sitting upright for prolonged periods because they experience dizzy spells due to insufficient blood pressure in the brain. When a quick change is made from a recumbent to a sitting position, momentary dizziness may be experienced because of a delay in the compensatory increase in arterial blood pressure, which occurs to provide an adequate supply of blood to the brain.

Standing is an important human evolutionary capacity, which has not yet reached perfection. Up to 20% of healthy young men faint when standing motionless for only twenty minutes because of blood pooling in the legs and abdomen (pulled down by gravity) and lack of blood supply to the brain. In most cases this happens when consciously trying to avoid movement, such as when standing at attention, an unnatural posture. Most people do not faint when standing in a relaxed position because the leg muscle action helps to pump the blood up against gravity. However, even relaxed standing cannot be tolerated by man for prolonged periods.

THE NEGATIVE-G CONDITION

What if we are under reverse gravity positions, i.e., a negative-g environment? This is when the head is lower than the feet in an inversely tilted position or completely upside down position. We may all have experienced this in our life. Untrained people cannot be upside down for long. It's unbearable. What about a tilted position? Depending on the degree of tilt, we may tolerate it for shorter or longer periods.

Despite the intolerance for a negative-g situation, we may gain some benefit too. From a common-sense point of view, we would guess that our heart beat will slow, our metabolic rate lower, the downward pulling of organs, fat, skin, etc., will be reversed to the opposite direction. There is a potential added benefit too. In fact, as we get older, our ability to fight against g-force is less. An older person suddenly moving from a head-down to a head-up position easily gets dizzy because blood cannot be sufficiently supplied to the head. An older person also has difficulty supplying enough blood to the head, causing deteriorating brain function. Similar to exercising muscles, a negative-g force may train our brain, hormones, and peripheral vascular systems to respond to g-force effectively even as we age. Thus, a negative-g force may enable us to live longer and look younger.

Winged birds typically outlive comparable sized land mammals. Bats outlive rats by a factor of four to six. Of the 4000 odd species of mammals on the earth, nearly one-quarter of them are bats. Are they a strong species because they live mostly horizontal or inverted? Or because they do not need to fight gravity as hard as the same size land mammal? Is it because bats sleep head down? Why are most ocean mammals ageless? Is it partially due to their near zero gravity environment?

There have been many studies about the negative-g conditions in the area of aerospace medicine in the 50's and 60's due to the advancement of space shuttles. The studies provide us much data on the hypothesis of the impact of negative-g on longevity.

Dr. Lawrence Lamb and Captain James Roman, USAF, performed a pioneering study published in the June 1961 volume of *Aerospace Medicine* on the circulatory response from +1g (in a normal standing position) to 0g (recumbent bed rest or weightlessness), and -1g force (in an upside-down position). A total of 224 subjects participated in the study. Under +1g, the sympathetic control of the circulatory system is stimulated. Through sympathetic influences, peripheral veins are contracted to restrict blood from pouring downward. Thus, peripheral resistance is maintained, which in turn provides for adequate distribution of cardiac output. This also increases heartbeat and blood pressure. When a sympathetic stimulation is dominant, it is common to see cardiac acceleration or an increased heart rate. In a recumbent position or bed rest, a transverse +1g force is acting on us, so it is a close approximation of a weightless situation for the circulatory system from head to feet. This will result in a cardiac system slowdown with slower heartbeat and relaxation of peripheral vascular resistance. In a head-down tilt situation simulating a negative-g, the heartbeat and peripheral vascular resistance is even more relaxed.

A study of hormonal response to a 10-degree head-down tilt (negative g-force) as compared to a standing position was conducted by Dr. Claude Gharib and others, published in the July 1988 and January 1992 issues of *Aerospace Medicine*. Under such a negative-g force, the contractility of the right heart (measured by the mean rate of right ventricular pressure) decreased by 34%, and the work performed reduced by 27%. There is a 15% progressive increase in plasma volume (more blood available) and an 18% decrease in diastolic blood pressure. There are also hormonal changes: plasma renin activity reduced by 60%, aldosterone by 63%, and catecholamines by 20%.

In summary, under a negative-g condition, metabolic rate and the downward compression of organs, skin, and spine are dramatically decreased. The head is supplied with ample blood to nourish its functioning. There is a strong hypothesis that a scientific negative-g therapy is critical to longevity.

METHODS TO ACHIEVE NEGATIVE-G

The scientific study of negative-g on longevity has never been proposed as far as we know. The belief in the benefit and the practice of this protocol are empirical.   It will be the reader's choice with the consultation of their physicians. We all have a limited lifetime. If we waited for 100% proof of scientific theory, we'd never try anything.   Based on the huge potential for reversing aging, we decided to present this to the reader.

There are several ways of practicing zero to negative g. For example, water sports. Since immersing in water provides a nice near zero g environment, most water sports are good for health, such as swimming and water aerobics.   Being in water is less stressful than equivalent land positions.   Another example is upside-down exercise. An ancient Chinese chi-gong practiced by the monks starts with a long period of standing upside down, using the hands as support. Gradually, one moves to a one-handed support and finally to one finger supporting the whole body. It was believed that this practice increases longevity. There are many other ways of being upside down, such as certain yoga postures, gymnastics exercises, and using tilt tables.

However, all these methods are limited because the time spent in daily or weekly exercises in a negative-g environment is very negligible as compared to a whole life span under constant pull of positive-g. In order to create a real impact, negative-g has to be a significant part of our life, rather than a one hour per week exercise.

APPLYING THE PROTOCOL

There is a breakthrough method to create such a negative-g environment for a significant portion of our lifetime. The authors have invented and practiced the *PingLongevity* Negative-g Therapy for the last five years.

Before presenting the method, we must stress again that all negative-g methods are based on empirical experience, as well as aerospace research oriented to the study of space shuttle physiology rather than longevity. Our readers are advised to consult with certified physicians before practicing *PingLongevity* Negative-g Therapy.

PingLongevity Negative-g Therapy. The idea is strikingly simple and the effect is dramatic. *If we are able to sleep every night on a tilted bed, head down, with a 10-20 degree angle, assuming an eight-hour sleep per day, we would have an equivalent 6-10% of our lifetime in a full negative 1g environment.* To be clear, for each 24-hour day, we would be spending an equivalent of 2.4 hours in a straight head-down feet-up position. Note that this therapy uses a straight tilted bed rather than beds that bend at the middle.

By using *PingLongevity* Negative-g Therapy, we can achieve 6-10% of a lifetime in a full negative 1g environment to counter the daily downward pull on organs, skin, and blood. In such a negative-g environment, we'd expect a slower heartbeat and lower blood pressure because the heart simply does not work as hard. Our real life five-year experience confirms this. It has been a lot easier to get into very deep sleep and rest.

In summary, negative-g therapy can be a significant part of life rather than an exercise with negligible duration. *PingLongevity* Negative-g Therapy is a breakthrough method to achieve 6-10% of full negative 1g environment during the entire lifetime. Be sure to consult with certified physicians before trying this method because of its limited scientific data in the area of anti-aging and risk evaluation.

EPILOGUE

We have attempted to give you what we have learned and experienced. In our lifetime journey, we continue to practice *PingLongevity* on our own body, mind, and spirit. We continue to explore the unlimited potentials of the human body and spirituality.

We know it is difficult to practice perfectly all seven protocols of *PingLongevity*. After all, each one of us has our own destination, fate, genes, and purpose in life. The fully achieved and developed are destined to be few. However, what about attaining 50%, 30%, or only 10% of what is required? Practicing even a fraction of *PingLongevity* will no doubt give you tremendous headroom for staying young longer and living healthier.

Our bodies, minds, and spirits are adaptive. The cleaner you are in body and spirit, the more you rid yourself of dirt. But it can go in the opposite direction, too. The more toxic you are, the more you crave toxins. We have seen our own preference in diet naturally change from junk food to super-clean, super-energized food. We have seen our spirits evolve from desiring an over-indulged material world to a spiritual world. We did not force ourselves. Our bodies wanted it. And your body probably does too. By choosing the right direction, your body will happily adapt.

Wouldn't it be nice to look and feel 10-30 years younger than you actually are? Wouldn't it be nice to be in your 40's, 50's, and 60's still full of youthful energy?

It's never too late, even if you have already been suffering from a degenerative disease of older age. You can reverse it. It's never too early either. Aging begins at puberty. You can preserve energy and stop aging.

We invite you to start the journey now. By joining us to make mankind healthier and more spiritually developed, we will all benefit together.

You can reach us at   www.pingclinic.com
pingclinic@pingclinic.com
1-866-608-1717 (for book orders)

Ping Wu
Taichi Tzu

GENERAL READINGS

Hayflick, Leonard, *How and Why We Age*, Ballantine Books, 1994.

Howell, Edward, *Food Enzymes for Health & Longevity*, Lotus Press, 1994.

Li, Yang, *I Ching and Traditional Chinese Medicine*, Beijing Sciences and Technology Press, 1997.

Liu, Yanchi, *The Essential Book of Traditional Chinese Medicine*, Columbia University Press, 1988.

Ni, Maoshing, *The Yellow Emperor's Classic of Medicine*, Shambhala, 1995.

Weindruch, Richard and Walford, Roy L., *The Retardation of Aging and Disease by Dietary Restriction*, Charles C. Thomas Publisher, 1988.

Wong, Eva, *Cultivating Stillness—A Taoist Manual for Transforming Body and Mind*, Shambhala, 1992.

INDEX

About the Authors

Ping Wu, M.D., is the founder of PingClinic. She was trained as a medical doctor in internal medicine in China and she received her master's degree in physiology from Boston University and her post-doctorate from the Cancer Research Center at the University of Arizona. She is an Arizona and California licensed acupuncturist and traditional Chinese medicine practitioner. PingClinic is located in Laguna Beach, California.

Taichi Tzu, Ph.D., is the inventor of the *PingLongevity* methods and seven protocols. He received his Ph.D. degree in applied sciences from Harvard University. He is a pioneering researcher in the combined methods of Taoist longevity, chi-gong, and modern anti-aging research.